MCQs for the FRCR Part 1

MCQs for the FRCR Part 1

by

Monica Khanna BSc (Hons) MBBS MRCS

Department of Clinical Radiology
Guy's and St Thomas' Hospitals
London

Leon Menezes MA BM BCh MRCP

Department of Clinical Radiology
Guy's and St Thomas' Hospitals
London

David Gallagher BSc MPhil CPhys MInst P

Department of Medical Physics
Guy's and St Thomas' Hospitals
London

GMM

Contents

Preface

This book is intended primarily for specialist registrars in clinical radiology who are sitting the first examination for the Fellowship of the Royal College of Radiologists. The multiple choice questions have been specifically arranged as practice papers, and have been written to reflect the number and style of the questions in the part one examination.

Anyone else who uses ionising radiation in their work will profit from studying this book, such as radiographers, nuclear physicians, and cardiologists.

Our aim is to help you pass the examination by testing your knowledge of the examination syllabus which covers the physics and regulations governing ionising radiation. This book will aid you greatly in refining your technique in answering negatively marked multiple choice questions as well as alerting you to areas of your knowledge that require further study. We hope the detailed answers will act as useful revision notes.

Good Luck!

M.K.
L.J.M.
D.G.
London, 2004

List of Abbreviations

ALARP   As low as reasonably practicable
ARSAC   Administration of radioactive substances advisory committee

CT   Computed tomography

DAP   Dose area product
DRL   Diagnostic reference level

ED   Effective dose
EMR   Electromagnetic radiation
ESD   Entrance surface dose

FOV   Field of view

GI   Gastro-intestinal
GP   General Practitioner
Gy   Gray

HSE   Health and Safety Executive
HVL   Half value layer

ICRP   International Commission on Radiological Protection
II   Image Intensifier
IRR   Ionising Radiation Regulations

MTF   Modulation transfer function
NHS   National Health Services

PET   Positron emission tomography

RPA   Radiation Protection Adviser
RPS   Radiation Protection Supervisor

SPECT   Single photon emission computed tomography
Sv   Sievert

TL   Thermoluminescent
TLD   Thermoluminescent dosimetry

W_R Radiation weighting factor
W_T Tissue weighting factor

Symbols, constants and definitions used in the text

A   =   mass number (number of neutrons plus protons in nucleus)
e   =   charge on the electron (1.6×10^{-19} C)
E   =   photon energy (J or eV)
E   =   Effective Dose (Sv)
eV   =   electron volt (1.6×10^{-19} J) (energy acquired by an electron when accelerated through 1 volt potential difference)
h =   Planck's constant (6.62×10^{-34} J.Hz^{-1})
f =   frequency (Hz)
N   =   Avogadro's number (6.02×10^{23})
Z   =   atomic number (number of protons in nucleus)
λ =   wavelength (m)
ρ =   mass density (kgm^{-3})
μ =   linear attenuation coefficient (m^{-1})
σ =   Compton linear attenuation coefficient (m^{-1})
τ =   Photoelectric linear attenuation coefficient (m^{-1})
Film γ =   Steepness of the characteristic curve

Gamma (γ) rays: electromagnetic radiation of nuclear origin

Kerma: Kinetic energy released per unit mass is the sum of the initial kinetic energies of charged ionising particles (or photons) released by incident uncharged particles (or photons) per unit mass of stopping medium.

X-rays: electromagnetic radiation produced in atomic orbital energy transitions

Section 1 – Questions

Q 1. Beta particles:

A. do contribute to patient absorbed dose
B. before coming to rest may travel in tissue for several millimetres
C. increase atomic number by one
D. change mass number in the nucleus
E. are emitted from the nucleus

Q 2. Electron capture:

A. occurs in neutron poor radionuclides
B. results in the emission of characteristic X-rays
C. the atomic number remains the same
D. the atomic mass number remains the same
E. ^{123}I decays wholly by electron capture

Q 3. The isotopes of an element have:

A. identical atomic numbers
B. identical atomic mass numbers
C. identical physical properties
D. identical chemical properties
E. the same density

Q 4. Radioactivity:

A. a radionuclide is an atom with an unstable nucleus
B. the activity of a radionuclide is the number of decays per hour
C. unit of activity is the Becquerel
D. radioactivity is a stochastic process
E. the daughter product is always radioactive

Q 5. **An increase in kilovoltage across an X-ray tube is associated with:**

A. a shortening of average wavelength of the X-ray spectrum
B. a relative increase in emitted X-ray intensity
C. an increase in penetration of the beam
D. a decrease in the half value layer of the beam
E. an increase in average frequency of the X-ray spectrum

Q 6. **The photoelectric effect in radiography:**

A. occurs about 70–80% of the time
B. is the interaction of a photon and a bound electron
C. occurs more frequently as the photon energy increases
D. interacts with the L-shell normally
E. is a pure absorption process in biological materials

Q 7. **Regarding Compton interactions:**

A. the scattered photon carries all the energy
B. all scatter is in a forward direction
C. they are responsible for 50% of interactions at 30 keV in soft tissues
D. the probability of interaction per mm length is proportional to the tissue density
E. the probability of interaction is proportional to the electron density

Q 8. **In a rotating anode X-ray tube:**

A. the anode is composed of a disc of pure tungsten for general radiography
B. the rotor has a blackened surface to increase radiation heat loss
C. an induction motor with a stator coil is used
D. the rotor bearings are lubricated with thin mineral oil
E. the molybdenum anode stem is designed to allow maximum heat conduction

Q 9. **In radiography the quality of the beam is changed by increasing:**

A. focus film distance
B. tube kilovoltage (kV)
C. exposure time
D. tube current (mA) with fixed kV
E. tube filtration

Q 10. **The amount of scattered radiation reaching the film in diagnostic X-ray imaging can be reduced by using:**

A. an air gap
B. a grid
C. beam collimation in the X-ray assembly to reduce field size
D. increased X-ray beam filtration
E. an increased tube potential between cathode and anode

Examination One

Questions

Q 11. Concerning mammography:

A. the maximum (peak) energy in the X-ray spectrum is determined by the characteristic radiation from molybdenum

B. a K-edge filter is used

C. the ideal radiation is 30 keV

D. typical mean glandular breast dose from a single film is 10 mGy

E. a focus to film distance of 100 cm is used

Q 12. Regarding deterministic effects of ionising radiation:

A. a threshold must be exceeded before an effect is observed

B. cataract induction is an example

C. the probability of a deterministic radiation effect is inversely proportional to dose

D. the severity of effect increases with radiation dose

E. genetic effects are somatic effects

Q 13. The duties of an employer under Ionising Radiation Regulations (IRR) (1999):

A. to ensure a Radiation Protection Adviser (RPA) advises the employer on the designation of controlled areas

B. to consult a RPA over the design of new installations

C. to set down local rules for the use of ionising radiation at work

D. to appoint a Radiation Protection Supervisor (RPS) where local rules are required

E. to ensure all persons to be classified, have a medical examination

14. Concerning IRR (1999):

  A. it is the responsibility of the employee to monitor and maintain the safety of equipment
  B. a controlled area is one in which doses are likely to exceed 30% of any dose limit for employees over 18 years of age
  C. dose limits are irrelevant when defining a supervised area
  D. controlled and supervised areas are defined in the systems of work
  E. local rules allow non-classified persons to enter a controlled area

Q 15. Regarding statutory responsibilities:

  A. the IRR (1999) are governed by the principle of as low as reasonably achievable
  B. IRMER (2000) lays down measures on the health protection of individuals against the dangers of ionising radiation in relation to medical exposure
  C. radioisotopes can only be administered by someone who holds a certificate of adequate training
  D. an administration of radioactive substances advisory committee (ARSAC) licence is granted to the health authority or trust
  E. crown immunity exempts all NHS hospitals in the UK from the regulations governing the storage of radioactive materials

Q 16. Concerning personal doses:

- **A.** workers who receive less than 30% of a dose limit cannot be classified
- **B.** a nurse who works permanently in an X-ray department is usually classified
- **C.** the radiation dose records of a classified worker must be kept for 2 years
- **D.** personal monitoring badges must be worn by all unclassified radiologists performing fluoroscopy
- **E.** the as low as reasonably practicable (ALARP) principle applies to occupational dose as well as patient dose

Q 17. Regarding radiation doses to patients and staff:

- **A.** under IRR (1999) the effective dose limit for members of the public is 1 mSv per annum
- **B.** a patient may receive approximately 4 mSv effective dose from an AP pelvis examination
- **C.** comforters and carers may receive 5 mSv over 5 years
- **D.** a member of staff may have to be classified if their effective dose looks likely to exceed 1 mSv per year
- **E.** the fatal cancer risk for an effective dose of 2 mSv is approximately 1 in 500,000 weighted over a population aged 18–60

Q 18. Film γ:

- **A.** is a plot of film latitude versus log exposure
- **B.** depends on emulsion crystal size
- **C.** increases with time of developing
- **D.** increases with temperature of developer
- **E.** low γ film is used in mammography

Q 19. Radiographic contrast can be increased by the following means:

A. compression of the region under examination
B. increasing the tube kilovoltage
C. use of a secondary radiation grid
D. increasing the area irradiated
E. use of intensifying screens

Q 20. Subject contrast is reduced if:

A. film γ is reduced
B. development time is too short
C. film is overexposed
D. kV is increased
E. size of beam is increased

Q 21. Regarding radiation dose to patients and members of the public:

A. the effective dose for a positron emission tomography (PET) head scan with ^{18}F-FDG is 5 mSv
B. the effective dose limit to the public is 1 mSv per annum
C. the background radiation dose is approximately 6 μSv per day
D. medical exposures contribute approximately 0.3 mSv on average per capita annually to UK collective dose
E. the entrance surface dose of a chest radiograph is 0.03 mGy

Q 22. Regarding image intensifiers:

   A. the limiting resolution can be measured with a line pair phantom
   B. the II input kerma rate at the image intensifier face is normally in the range of $0.2–1.0\,\mu Gys^{-1}$ during fluoroscopy
   C. the output phosphor is made out of caesium iodide
   D. brightness gain is the sum of flux gain and minification gain
   E. measured spatial resolution is usually poor on magnified fields of view

Q 23. Concerning a digital image intensifier and TV system:

   A. the TV camera is the limiting factor on the system's spatial resolution
   B. film screen resolution is poorer than image resolution in fluoroscopy
   C. frame averaging images can reduce the effects of quantum noise
   D. the focus skin distance should be preferably not less than 45 cm on stationary imaging equipment
   E. energy imparted to the patient cannot be estimated with a dose area product meter positioned on the tube beam port

Q 24. Radiopharmaceuticals used for diagnostic imaging should ideally:

   A. emit photons with an energy greater than 300 keV
   B. have a physical half-life of more than 4 days
   C. decay to a stable state
   D. be a pure γ emitter
   E. be stable in vivo

In computed tomography (CT):

   A. third generation scanners rotate detector array and tube
   B. xenon gas can be used as a detector
   C. slice width affects spatial resolution
   D. tube anode/cathode axis is perpendicular to the detector array
   E. as slice thickness increases, the partial volume effect tends to decrease

Q 1. **Beta particles:**

A. are light charged particles
B. are ionising
C. β− decay occurs in neutron poor nuclides
D. β+ decay occurs in neutron rich nuclides
E. have a charge of e

Q 2. **The nucleus of every atom contains:**

A. a neutron
B. a proton
C. a positron
D. a photon
E. an electron

Q 3. **Regarding radioactivity:**

A. a fixed number of atoms decay per unit time
B. effective half-life is always shorter than biological or physical half-lives
C. the energy is characteristic of the radionuclide
D. iodine-131 emits β particles
E. radioactive decay depends on temperature

Q 4. The photoelectric effect:

A. is an interaction between an incident photon and loosely bound electron

B. causes the irradiated atom to be ionised

C. shows a general increase with increased photon energy of the X-ray beam

D. is an important mode of attenuation in diagnostic radiology

E. is independent of atomic number

Q 5. Compton scattering:

A. is the collision of a photon with a tightly bound K-shell electron

B. results in increased energy loss with increased angle of scatter of the photon

C. is unaffected by the electron density of the scattering medium

D. is an insignificant process in image formation in diagnostic radiology

E. becomes less significant for imaging at greater energies

Q 6. The spectrum obtained from an X-ray tube:

A. has a maximum energy determined by the peak tube potential (kVp)

B. depends on the target material

C. varies with distance from the anode to cathode

D. is affected by filtration

E. varies with tube current

Q 7. In comparison to the single phase generator, a three phase generator:

A. is more commonly found in older X-ray systems
B. provides greater output for the same radiographic factors
C. gives a reduced skin dose to the patient for the same exposure
D. allows a shorter exposure time
E. is always required for use with a high speed rotating anode tube

Q 8. The radiation output (measured at the entrance surface of the patient) from an X-ray tube increases with:

A. increasing kilovoltage
B. increasing tube current
C. increasing atomic number of the target
D. the use of filters
E. increased distance to the patient

Q 9. X-rays are produced in an X-ray tube as a result of interactions between:

A. moving protons and target electrons
B. moving protons and target protons
C. moving electrons and target nuclei
D. moving neutrons and target nuclei
E. moving electrons and inner shell target electrons

Q 10. Regarding the use of compression in mammography:

A. a smaller volume of breast tissue is irradiated
B. less scatter results
C. fewer structures are overlying one another
D. a film of narrow latitude is needed
E. is always used unless it is not tolerated

Examination Two

Questions

MCQs MCQs for the FRCR Part 1

15

Q 11. With deterministic effects the following are true:

A. there is a threshold above which there is no effect
B. the threshold dose is constant for different pathological reactions
C. the severity of effect is dose dependent
D. if there is full recovery of the patient, then effects are non-additive
E. the probability of effects occurring depends on dose

Q 12. Dose measured or calculated at depth in the patient:

A. increases when tube potential increases but optical density is kept constant
B. decreases when tube potential increases but mAs product remains the same
C. increases when filtration decreases, all other factors being equal
D. is completely independent of entrance field size at the patient surface
E. is dependent on focal spot size, all other factors being equal

Q 13. A whole body bimonthly dosimeter reading of 7 mSv was recorded by a female member of staff in the radiology department. In accordance with IRR (1999), the following should happen:

A. an investigation should be carried out immediately
B. the Health and Safety Executive (HSE) should be notified
C. she should immediately become a classified worker
D. the member of staff should have a medical examination
E. the member of staff should stop working with ionising radiation immediately

Q 14. **Concerning radiation protection:**

    A. Radiation Protection Advisers normally reside in an X-ray department

    B. the radiation protection committee should have a representative of the hospital management in it

    C. a General Practitioner (GP) who requests a chest radiograph is clinically directing the examination

    D. a radiographer who performs a chest X-ray acts as a practitioner under the IRMER Regulations

    E. during pacemaker wire insertion, the radiographer authorises the exposure

Q 15. **Regarding the Medicines (Administration of Radioactive Substances) Regulations:**

    A. procedures can only be carried out by an ARSAC certificate holder

    B. the application for an ARSAC certificate has to be signed by a Radiation Protection Adviser

    C. an ARSAC certificate is usually valid for 10 years

    D. the ARSAC certificate holder is responsible for discharging patients from the Nuclear Medicine department

    E. the maximum dose to the patient is defined in the ARSAC certificate by the half-life of the radiopharmaceutical

Q 16. **Concerning annual whole body doses:**

    A. most health workers receive less than 3 mSv per year

    B. for radiographers are usually higher than for radiologists

    C. for radiologists are usually higher than for cardiologists

    D. limits are defined in IRR (1999) for patients while undergoing radiographic examination

    E. patients in an X-ray department waiting area are regarded as members of the public

Q 17. Concerning diagnostic reference levels:

A. are always measured in mSv
B. are set nationally
C. represent dose limits
D. are different for different ages of patient
E. are set for each piece of equipment

Q 18. Regarding staff and patient dosimetry:

A. a dose area product (DAP) meter should be placed between the patient and the film
B. the skin entry dose for a lateral lumbar spine is usually more than that of a plain abdomen film
C. examinations of the limbs and joints make up over 10% of the collective dose from medical radiation
D. the mean annual effective dose for medical workers is typically less than 0.2 mSv
E. a single fraction of 2 Gy may cause a transient erythema which would be expected to be maximum at 24 h

Q 19. Gadolinium oxysulphide screens:

A. increase unsharpness relative to calcium tungstate screens
B. are faster than non-screen film
C. display increased speed with increased crystal size
D. their speed increases with increased thickness
E. have relatively little effect on film/screen γ compared to non-screen film

Q 20. Unsharpness:

A. is decreased with the use of a screen
B. increases with increased kVp
C. decreases with increased film object distance
D. decreases with increased tube patient distance
E. is decreased with the use of fine grain films

Q 21. With image intensifiers, brightness gain:

    A. increases with increase in voltage across the intensifier

    B. increases with decrease in the output phosphor size

    C. is increased by the use of a calcium tungstate input phosphor

    D. is increased by increasing the exposure to the input phosphor

    E. is increased by the use of the horizontal position

Q 22. The zinc-cadmium-sulphide output phosphor in an image intensifier:

    A. absorbs only a small percentage of the X-rays

    B. has a lot of afterglow

    C. emits a blue light

    D. the eye is sensitive to its emissions

    E. has an intensification factor of 2

Q 23. In carrying out quality control tests of X-ray equipment:

    A. kV can be measured with a film sensitometer

    B. timer accuracy is measured with an ion chamber

    C. a spatial resolution of 12 lp/cm would be acceptable for a fluoroscopic barium examination

    D. at 80 kV, a half value layer (HVL) of 2.8 mm Al would indicate adequate filtration

    E. film/screen contact is tested with a resolution grid inside the cassette

Q 24. In radionuclide imaging, effective dose is:

A. 18 mSv for an 80 MBq cardiac thallium scan on an adult patient
B. inversely proportional to the administered radioactivity
C. dependent on the γ emission probability per disintegration
D. dependent on the biological half-life of the nuclide
E. independent of image acquisition time

Q 25. Spatial resolution in CT depends on:

A. slice thickness
B. slice spacing
C. pixel size
D. window level
E. matrix size

Q 1. Concerning atomic structure:

A. the outer shell electrons are termed valence electrons

B. the transition between L and K or M and K-shell, gives rise to the emission of characteristic radiation

C. the atomic number is the number of nucleons

D. the mass number is always equal to the number of protons

E. the atomic number equals the number of electrons in a neutral non-ionised atom

Q 2. Regarding the electromagnetic radiation spectrum:

A. X-rays have a higher frequency than visible light

B. a wavelength of 532 nm corresponds to green light

C. an X-ray and γ-ray photon of the same energy can be distinguished

D. an electromagnetic quantum has energy inversely proportional to its wavelength

E. electromagnetic radiation includes Auger emission

Q 3. Regarding an X-ray tube:

A. a low tube potential always suffices with a stationary anode

B. a decrease in filament current tends to reduce the tube output

C. a decrease in tube potential reduces the output of the tube

D. a rotating anode X-ray tube for general use is not made of a tungsten-rhenium alloy

E. heat production in the tube is of the order of 98%

Q 4. The output from a diagnostic X-ray tube:

A. can be increased by an increase in the filtration
B. is reduced by lowering the kVp
C. depends on the anode material
D. is proportional to the tube current
E. is inversely proportional to the focal spot size

Q 5. The intensity of the radiation from an X-ray tube at a given point in the primary beam depends on the:

A. tube current (mA)
B. atomic number of the target material
C. distance between the cathode and anode
D. thickness of the added filtration
E. distance from the target

Q 6. Added tube filtration:

A. decreases the intensity of the X-ray beam
B. is usually made of copper for diagnostic tubes
C. increases the skin dose to the patient
D. changes the quality of the emergent X-ray beam
E. should be sufficient to give a total filtration equivalent to 2.5 mm aluminium for a diagnostic tube operating up to 150 kVp

Q 7. Regarding X-ray attenuation in materials:

A. the half value thickness of a material is inversely proportional to its linear attenuation coefficient
B. the photoelectric effect predominates in soft tissue above 30 keV
C. photoelectric interactions in soft tissue, give rise to characteristic radiation of such low energy, that it can be considered locally absorbed at the site of interaction
D. the Compton linear attenuation coefficient σ reduces with increasing photon energy E
E. the high contrast seen in CT, is not due to the photoelectric effect

Q 8. Regarding scattered radiation:

A. the larger the field size, the less scattered radiation will be produced
B. the air gap technique increases the amount of scattered radiation reaching the image receptor
C. the amount of scattered radiation reaching the image receptor decreases as tube potential increases
D. forward scatter predominates at over 30 kVp
E. the ratio of primary to scattered radiation may be as low as 0.1 in diagnostic radiology

Q 9. In an imaging system for mammography:

A. an X-ray tube with a rhodium target and filtration can be used
B. a focal spot size of greater than 0.5 mm is advised to allow greater tube currents and reduce exposure times
C. a single sided emulsion is never used
D. tube potential in the range 17–19 keV is normally selected
E. the heel effect must be minimised in mammography tube design

Q 10. Regarding quality assurance of diagnostic X-ray equipment:

A. kVp accuracy should be checked at least annually
B. Leeds test objects may be used to measure tube output
C. poor film screen contact produces uneven blackening of the film
D. focal spot size may be measured using a star test object
E. kVp accuracy of $\pm 10\,kV$ is acceptable

Q 11. The dose to a patient may be reduced when using a film screen system by:

A. selecting a lower receptor dose on the automatic exposure control for a given tube potential
B. reducing beam filtration
C. removing any compression band present
D. decreasing the object to film distance
E. using a low ratio grid

Q 12. A stochastic radiation effect is one in which:

A. there is a threshold dose level below which no effects occur
B. the severity of the effect varies with dose
C. the probability of the effect occurring varies with dose
D. cataract of the lens is an example
E. leukaemia is an example

Q 13. In radiation protection:

A. stochastic effects are defined as biological effects whose incidence is proportional to the dose, provided a threshold is exceeded

B. the dose equivalent is the same as the equivalent dose

C. a classified worker is someone who has attended a 'core of knowledge' course and is therefore trained in the use of ionising radiation

D. stochastic and genetic effects always occur when tissues are irradiated

E. local rules are to allow for circumstances where radiation exposure could occur

Q 14. Equivalent dose is a quantity that:

A. is averaged over all tissues of the body

B. uses a radiation weighting factor to account for differences in biological effectiveness of different types of radiation

C. is used to set occupational dose organ limits

D. has the same weighting factor for X-rays and γ-rays

E. is measured in Sieverts (Sv)

Q 15. Ionisation in air or in air equivalent material is commonly used to measure the quantity of radiation because:

A. air has a similar atomic number to muscle tissue

B. because the effects of changes in temperature and pressure are small, they can normally be ignored in diagnostic radiology dosimetry

C. ionisation currents are large enough to be measured with a simple ampmeter

D. free air chambers can be made very compact and simple to use

E. because the IRR (1999) states that it must be used

Q 16. IRR (1999) states the following dose limits:

A. 5 mSv to the whole body of a member of the public
B. 150 mSv to the lens of the eye of a radiologist
C. 50 mSv to the individual organs or tissues of a radiographer
D. 10 mSv during any consecutive three-month period to the abdomen of a woman of reproductive capacity
E. 20 mSv per year averaged over 5 years, but no more than 50 mSv in a single year, to the whole body of a radiology department assistant

Q 17. Radiation legislation requires:

A. all persons working with radiation to have their personal doses monitored
B. all radiation workers to receive a whole body dose of less than 20 mSv per annum
C. a controlled area to be defined only if the instantaneous dose rates exceed 7.5 μSv per hour
D. patient doses to be below certain prescribed limits
E. the employer to be responsible for ensuring that patient doses are ALARP

Q 18. Regarding radiation safety in nuclear medicine, when administering doses to patients:

A. portable scintillation monitor is not suitable for the measurement of personal contamination from electron capture nuclides
B. when drawing up injections finger doses may be reduced by keeping the active bolus in a syringe away from the fingers
C. radioactive solutions of low specific activity may be pipetted by mouth
D. because of the short half-life of all nuclides, spills may be left to decay safely
E. 0.25 mm lead aprons will provide effective protection against 140 keV photons

Q 19. The speed of a film/screen combination is affected by the:

A. energy of the incident X-ray
B. thickness of the screen
C. shape of the film grains
D. atomic number of the screen material
E. developer temperature

Q 20. The following statements about film/screen combinations are true:

A. the shape of the characteristic curve is largely determined by the properties of the film
B. increasing the developer temperature increases the saturation density of the film
C. less than 10% of the film density is due to the direct effect of the X-rays on the film
D. the use of high kV techniques increases the latitude
E. phosphors with a high X-ray to light conversion efficiency reduce noise

Q 21. In a scintillation detector using a NaI crystal:

A. the efficiency depends on the thickness of the crystal
B. the output pulse from the photomultiplier tube is dependent on the energy of the γ-ray detected
C. high energy β particles are detected
D. the NaI crystal is hygroscopic
E. a collimator is used to reduce scatter

Q 22. Concerning radioactivity in a generator:

    A. activity of 1 MBq = 1 disintegration per second
    B. the daughter always decays with the same activity as the parent when in equilibrium
    C. the activity is independent of the half-life of the daughter
    D. the daughter decays exponentially when at equilibrium
    E. the activity is not related to the time between elutions

Q 23. In a parent-daughter radionuclide generator, the amount of activity of the daughter at equilibrium:

    A. is constant
    B. is dependent on the volume of the element
    C. is much less than the activity of the parent
    D. is independent of the half-life of the daughter
    E. is independent of the time since the column was last eluted

Q 24. The modulation transfer function:

    A. expresses the ratio of the recorded information to the available information in the X-ray beam
    B. reflects the information lost when X-rays are recorded
    C. of a system only depends on its resolution
    D. may be derived from Fourier analysis
    E. does not allow comparison of alternative imaging systems

Q **25. In computed tomography:**

    A. the pixel value represents the linear attenuation coefficient in a voxel

    B. Compton interactions predominate in the patient

    C. 5 mm copper filtration is required

    D. fat has a typical value of -100 Hounsfield units

    E. narrowing of the window width decreases contrast in the processed image

Q 1. Beta particles:

A. are associated with nuclear decay

B. are not associated with a change in mass number during radioactive decay

C. increase atomic number by one during radioactive decay

D. contribute to patient absorbed dose

E. may travel for a few metres in air if energetic

Q 2. The following statements are true concerning X-ray spectra:

A. characteristic X-rays contribute more to a mammography tube target spectrum than they do with a general radiography tube

B. very few X-rays less than 10 keV are created at the target

C. X-ray spectra used in CT usually have a higher effective energy than those used in fluoroscopy

D. the shape of the bremsstrahlung spectrum is a strong function of the design of the focusing cup at the filament

E. the X-ray spectrum can be measured using a scintillation detector

Q 3. The diagnostic X-ray tube:

A. never produces a monoenergetic X-ray spectrum if operated with a K-edge absorption filter the same as the target material

B. a fixed rather than rotating anode system is used on all mobile image intensifier systems

C. on broad focus emits more photons per mm² compared to fine focus

D. tube replacement may not be required for some years

E. higher anode spin speeds are required on mobiles because of higher tube loading

Q 4. The effect of a grid is to:

A. increase the dose resulting from scattered radiation to the patient

B. reduce the radiographic contrast

C. decrease the necessary exposure

D. decrease the penetration of the radiation

E. increase the scattered radiation reaching the film

Q 5. Assuming image receptor dose remains constant, additional beam filtration of an X-ray beam:

A. decreases the mean photon energy of the beam

B. decreases the half value thickness

C. increases the skin entrance surface dose (ESD)

D. decreases the dose to the superficial tissues

E. decreases the radiographic contrast in the image receptor

Q 6. **For a given set of exposure factors the scatter around a patient is:**

A. increased by calcium tungstate screens as opposed to rare earth screens
B. increased by increasing the radiation beam size
C. increased by increasing the filtration
D. decreased by increasing the focus to film distance
E. less backwards than forwards

Q 7. **The effective focal spot size of a rotating anode tube is influenced by:**

A. the angle of slope of the anode
B. the size of the filament
C. the speed of anode rotation
D. the diameter of the anode disc
E. the anode film distance

Q 8. **The following statements are true when using the air gap technique in PA chest radiography:**

A. wide angled scattered radiation misses the film
B. slow intensifying screens are required
C. the focus to film distance must be increased
D. radiographic kV must be lower than with conventional chest radiography
E. the air gap must be at least 30 cm

Q 9. **In mammography:**

A. a focal spot of 0.5 mm should be used for magnification
B. palladium is used as a target material
C. the use of compression reduces patient dose
D. the anode heel effect is useful
E. a stationary grid is used in preference to a moving grid

Q 10. Increasing the tube potential from 60 to 80 would be expected to have the following effects:

A. require the use of a $CaWO_4$ screen
B. increase the relative number of photoelectric interactions in the patient
C. reduce the film contrast
D. increase the radiation dose to the patient, for the same image receptor dose
E. require the mAs to be reduced to approximately 32% of its previous value to achieve the same image receptor dose

Q 11. The entrance surface dose rate measured at the beam entry point on the patient's skin:

A. decreases with field size
B. decreases with the current flowing between cathode and anode
C. is proportional to the atomic number (Z) of the target
D. varies as the square of the focal spot to patient distance
E. varies with the amount of filtration used in the beam

Q 12. Geometrical unsharpness is decreased if the:

A. effective focal spot is decreased in size
B. film-focus distance decreases
C. object to film distance increases
D. patient movement is captured on the image
E. exposure time is too short

Q 13. The term grid ratio is:

    A. the height of the lead slots compared to the area of the grid

    B. the exposure time with the grid divided by the exposure time without it

    C. the attenuation in the lead compared to the attenuation in the interspace material

    D. a measure of the ability of the grid to stop primary radiation

    E. related to the thickness of the grid compared to the area of the grid

Q 14. Typical examples of non-stochastic effects of radiation include:

    A. genetic effects

    B. fibrosis

    C. leukaemia

    D. cataracts

    E. decreased sperm production

Q 15. Thermoluminescent dosimetry (TLD) is an important dosimetric method because:

    A. ionisation in thermoluminescent materials results in electrons being trapped

    B. thermoluminescent material can be made in a range of sizes

    C. TLD has a precision better than 1%

    D. it does not require independent calibration

    E. it is unaffected by temperature over a very wide range

Q 16. Quantum mottle can be reduced by:

A. developing the film longer
B. using a longer X-ray exposure
C. using a thicker intensifying screen
D. raising the temperature of the developer
E. by exposing the film twice

Q 17. The following contribute to film fog formation:

A. the construction of the cassette used
B. the dye used in the base
C. the support provided for the phosphor in the screen
D. the binder used in the intensifying screen
E. the duration of the developing process

Q 18. During film processing:

A. the film γ may be affected
B. the temperature is closely related to the optical density
C. the processing time tends to be constant across all types of film
D. the developer does not reduce silver bromide in the image
E. the fixer does not harden the emulsion

Q 19. In a caesium iodide image intensifier system:

A. limiting spatial resolution of 20 line pairs per mm at the output phosphor may be expected
B. contrast is dependent on the image intensifier input diameter
C. the image intensifier's input dose rate reduces when selecting magnified fields
D. the minimum visible detail size is smaller on plain film radiographs than in the fluoroscopic image
E. the measured patient maximum ESD should not exceed 100 mGy/min

Q 20. Regarding staff protection:

A. the heaviest tolerable lead apron should be worn
B. aprons have a lead equivalent of 1.25 to 1.5 mm
C. lead aprons afford adequate protection from the primary beam
D. lead gloves afford adequate protection from the primary beam
E. a standard lead apron will transmit less than 10% of the incident dose at 100 kV

Q 21. Under IRR (1999), an employee must become a classified worker if:

A. the dose to their eyes is likely to exceed 150 mSv annually
B. they are likely to receive an annual effective dose greater than 6 mSv
C. four-tenths of a relevant dose limit is exceeded
D. they work in different locations
E. they become pregnant

Q 22. Under IRMER (2000), the following are true regarding 'referrers':

A. only doctors and dentists are permitted to request an X-ray
B. they can request anything from 'Making Best Use of a Department of Clinical Radiology'
C. their identities must be kept by the employer
D. they must provide sufficient relevant clinical information to allow justification of the exposure
E. they must be adequately trained

Q 23. In the following circumstances the Health and Safety Executive (HSE) must be notified:

A. dose exceeding investigation level
B. medical exposure much greater than intended
C. loss or theft of a radioactive source
D. release or spillage leading to significant contamination
E. failure to follow work instructions and local rules

Q 24. In radionuclide imaging the radiation dose to the patient is:

A. dependent on the energy of the γ photon emissions
B. inversely proportional to the administered radioactivity
C. dependent on the biological half-life of the radiopharmaceutical
D. usually greater than 20 mSv for a patient undergoing a Thallium-201 myocardial scan
E. dependent on the image acquisition time

Q 25. The effective dose in CT of the abdomen will be reduced by:

A. increasing the spacing between slices
B. increasing the mA, other factors remaining constant
C. increasing the number of detectors
D. using spiral scanning rather than selective scanning
E. decreasing the field of view

Q 1. In a Compton interaction:

A. the smaller the angle through which the photon is scattered the more energy it loses

B. there is an interaction between a photon and a bound electron resulting in the emission of an Auger electron

C. the frequency change of the photon depends on the atomic number of the scattering material

D. lower energy photons tend to lose a smaller fraction of their initial energy than higher energy photons

E. the number of scatter interactions in a given sample is proportional to the electron density of the scattering medium

Q 2. The photoelectric effect:

A. produces the emission of characteristic radiation

B. for the same photon energy will occur more frequently in lead than aluminium

C. produces scatter

D. predominates when X-rays interact with barium

E. predominates in CT

Q 3. Regarding the Compton effect in diagnostic radiology:

A. it is the greatest source of attenuation in fat for photons above 30 keV

B. photons retain most of their energy

C. for a given energy more interactions will occur in the same volume of soft tissue compared to bone

D. it is proportional to electron density

E. it depends upon atomic number

Q 4. **The effect of X-ray scattering:**

A. recorded on the film can be reduced by the use of a lower kVp
B. is to reduce contrast in a film
C. is to reduce the optical density in a film
D. is to reduce the apparent attenuation in an anatomical structure
E. in the patient leads to larger staff eye doses in over-couch tube fluoroscopy units

Q 5. **Using an ionisation chamber the output of an X-ray unit has been measured:**

A. the half value thickness of the beam will not be affected as the chamber is air equivalent
B. the output will depend on the filtration but not the mA
C. the output will change with the filtration and the kVp
D. the output will change with the mAs and distance
E. the output will change if a larger ionisation chamber is connected to the same electrometer (the device used to measure the charge created in the chamber)

Q 6. **Increasing the tube potential applied to an X-ray tube increases the:**

A. mAs setting required to produce a radiograph of unit optical density
B. radiation dose measured at a given distance per mAs
C. entrance surface dose to produce a radiograph of acceptable density
D. amount of scattered radiation reaching the image receptor
E. attenuation of the X-ray beam in the patient

Q 7. X-ray beam collimation:

- **A.** decreases the beam intensity
- **B.** decreases contrast in the image
- **C.** increases the radiation exposure of the patient
- **D.** increases the amount of scatter produced in the patient
- **E.** does not affect geometric unsharpness

Q 8. Radiographic image contrast is improved by:

- **A.** not using a grid
- **B.** using less beam filtration
- **C.** using an intensifying screen
- **D.** using a carbon fibre table top
- **E.** increasing the kVp

Q 9. Geometrical unsharpness is increased by using:

- **A.** a greater object to film distance
- **B.** a longer exposure time
- **C.** an anti-scatter grid
- **D.** a decreased focus to object distance
- **E.** a decreased target angle

Q 10. A high kV radiographic technique:

- **A.** suppresses bony detail in the image
- **B.** results in a lower radiation dose to the patient (for a given optical density)
- **C.** results in improved contrast
- **D.** has disadvantages in barium examinations
- **E.** is suitable for use in conventional tomography

Q 11. The amount of scattered radiation relative to the primary beam, reaching the film may be reduced by:

A. decreasing the tube current (mA)
B. increasing the beam size
C. using high definition screen in preference to a high speed screen
D. decreasing the tube filtration
E. increasing patient thickness

Q 12. Radiographic contrast is affected by:

A. tube potential
B. focal spot size
C. film/screen γ
D. subject contrast
E. focus to film distance

Q 13. Regarding radiation doses:

A. the average annual effective dose to the UK population from medical exposures is 300 μSv
B. the effective dose limit for members of the public is 6 mSv per annum
C. the average annual natural background radiation dose in UK is approximately 6 μSv
D. the entrance surface dose is approximately 0.2 mGy for a chest radiograph
E. a SPECT Tc-99m bone scan administering 800 MBq to a patient, results in an effective dose of 5 mSv

Q 14. Barium enema patient doses can be reduced by:

A. using an over couch X-ray tube fluoroscopy system
B. a carbon fibre patient table
C. acquiring images using digital fluorography rather than conventional film
D. using magnification
E. low pulse rate digital fluoroscopy

Q 15. Under IRR (1999) an employer is responsible for:

    A. instruction and training of employees

    B. designating controlled areas

    C. ensuring doses are within dose limits

    D. appointing a Radiation Protection Adviser

    E. replacing personal protective equipment every 12 months

Q 16. The Radiation Protection Supervisor:

    A. must be medically qualified

    B. distributes and collects dosimeters used by staff

    C. enables employer to ensure local rules are being followed

    D. investigates overexposures

    E. must be qualified in medical physics

Q 17. Regarding IRMER (2000):

    A. overall responsibility for keeping dose to the patient as low as reasonably practicable rests with the practitioner

    B. the practitioner is the only person entitled to authorise an X-ray exposure

    C. the practitioner is the only person entitled to justify an X-ray exposure

    D. practitioners are trained experts in medical physics

    E. practitioners may be operators

Q 18. Concerning intensifying screens:

    A. the main emission of La_2OBr is green light

    B. rare earth phosphor speed is independent of tube potential (kVp)

    C. the main emission of Gd_2O_2S phosphor is blue light

    D. high frequency radiation is absorbed and emitted as low frequency radiation

    E. $CaWO_4$ requires no activator

Q 19. Intensifying screens:

    A. decrease the sharpness of a radiograph

    B. increase the exposure required by a factor of 10 or more

    C. increase the film speed

    D. emit visible light

    E. increase radiographic contrast

Q 20. Concerning noise in an X-ray image:

    A. noise is increased by using a screen with a high light conversion efficiency

    B. noise is increased by using a phosphor with a decreased absorption coefficient

    C. visibility of low contrast objects is reduced by noise

    D. increasing phosphor thickness decreases noise

    E. noise occurs more commonly with rare earth screens due to their increased efficiency compared to $CaWO_4$ screens

Q 21. In a γ camera:

    A. spatial resolution is of the order of 1 lp/mm

    B. the pulse height analyser enables two radionuclides to be distinguished from one another

    C. a thicker crystal improves spatial resolution

    D. photoelectric interactions predominate in the crystal for 140 keV photons

    E. the main function of a collimator is to absorb scattered photons

Q 22. The following statements are true:

    A. ^{99m}Tc has a photon energy of 140 keV

    B. ^{99m}Tc has a physical half-life of 6 days

    C. ^{18}F has a physical half-life of 6 h

    D. ^{99m}Tc is a daughter product of the parent radionuclide ^{99}Mo

    E. ^{18}F is produced in a cyclotron

A. the crystal and collimator are changed to suit the resolution and sensitivity required
B. the collimator provides the best method of improving contrast
C. the resolution is improved by placing the camera as close as possible to the patient
D. spatial resolution is improved by taking a tomographic view
E. the most important consideration when choosing an isotope is that its decay energy should be between 100 and 300 keV

Q 24. **In computed tomography:**

A. spatial resolution is improved by decreasing the pixel size
B. noise will be reduced if the slice thickness is increased
C. each detector has its own collimator
D. a xenon gas detector is more efficient than a thallium doped NaI detector
E. photoelectric interactions predominate in the patient

Q 25. **In computed tomography:**

A. spatial resolution improves with an increase in matrix size
B. spatial resolution is superior to plain radiography
C. small quantities of calcium can have a significant effect on partial volume averaging in a voxel
D. noise is independent of slice width
E. the ability to detect low contrast details depends more on object size than pixel size in the image

Examination Five

Questions

Q 1. The nucleus of an atom:

A. contains protons
B. is not involved in the Compton scattering event
C. can be made unstable by irradiating it with a diagnostic X-ray beam
D. is the source of γ-rays
E. is 10^{-15} m in diameter

Q 2. The photoelectric interaction:

A. is an interaction between an atomic electron and an incident X-ray
B. leads to approximately 50% absorption of the incident photon energy
C. is more likely to result in the production of characteristic X-rays if the atomic number of the material is high
D. in lead gives rise to an absorption edge at 35 keV
E. is more likely to occur in soft tissue than bone

Q 3. In diagnostic X-ray production:

A. most of the energy used is converted into ionising radiation
B. the line focus principle is used to increase tube loading
C. target heating is a limiting factor
D. bremsstrahlung radiation results from the interaction between cathode electrons and target material
E. the heel effect occurs on the cathode side of the central axis of the X-ray beam

Q 4. The rating of a tube in diagnostic radiology:

A. is a measure of the maximum mA that can be used for given values of kV, focal spot size and exposure time
B. is higher for half wave rectification than full wave rectification
C. is higher for a rotating anode than stationary anode
D. is greater for a smaller focal spot
E. is limited by heat production

Q 5. Regarding high kilovoltage techniques:

A. result in increased tube heating
B. result in decreased patient dose
C. lower tube loading will allow more frequent use of a fine focus
D. in chest radiography uses an air gap
E. in chest radiography is used to visualise bony detail

Q 6. The secondary electrons produced by X-rays are responsible for:

A. biological effects
B. thermal effects
C. induced radioactivity
D. ionisation
E. photographic properties

Q 7. In mammography:

A. compression is used to improve the contrast
B. K-edge filters are not used
C. Compton scattering is the dominant interaction in the patient
D. a minimum spatial resolution of 10 lp/mm is required
E. the focal spot size is 300 microns

Q 8. The air gap technique:

- **A.** uses a gap between the grid and the detector to reduce the scatter at the detector
- **B.** is most effective with larger gaps
- **C.** produces a minified image
- **D.** is used in CT imaging to prevent scatter reaching the detector array
- **E.** is used in chest radiography

Q 9. The induction of cancer following exposure to ionising radiation:

- **A.** has a threshold of 20 mSv
- **B.** is an effect, the severity of which increases with dose
- **C.** is an effect, the probability of which increases with dose
- **D.** carries a 1 in 17,000 risk of inducing fatal cancer per mSv
- **E.** may be caused by DNA damage and subsequent chromosome aberrations

Q 10. Dose can be reduced by using a:

- **A.** grid
- **B.** short film focus distance
- **C.** small focal spot
- **D.** fast film/screen combination
- **E.** low kVp

Q 11. Concerning the effects of ionising radiation:

    A. transient skin erythema occurs above a single dose of 2 Sv

    B. the lens of the eye is more radiosensitive than the cornea

    C. there is a potential for severe mental retardation following irradiation in the third trimester

    D. the radiation weighting factor for electrons is the same as for positrons

    E. the likelihood of Down's syndrome is increased by irradiation in the first trimester

Q 12. Regarding dosimetry:

    A. one gray is defined as an energy deposition of one joule per medium by any type of radiation

    B. the effective dose equivalent takes into account the effect that radiation has on different organs

    C. a stochastic effect describes the probability of the occurrence of a harmful effect of radiation

    D. the effective dose limit for a worker is an average 20 mSv per annum

    E. using a constant potential kV waveform results in a higher patient dose for the same exposure

Q 13. An employee must become a classified worker if:

    A. they work more than five sessions a week with ionising radiation

    B. 3/10 of a relevant dose limit is likely to be exceeded

    C. they are likely to get an effective dose greater than 6 mSv annually

    D. the hand dose may exceed 150 mSv per annum

    E. they become pregnant

Q 14. Under IRR (1999), designated areas:

    A. are so called by the employer
    B. are supervised areas where a person is likely to receive at least 1/10 of an employee dose limit
    C. are controlled areas where a person is likely to receive 5 mSv
    D. need not be signposted
    E. local rules do not apply

Q 15. Under IRMER (2000), concerning diagnostic reference levels:

    A. diagnostic reference levels should be established for all procedures
    B. the employer will review when diagnostic reference levels are exceeded
    C. the dose for every medical exposure must be recorded
    D. the diagnostic reference level is set at the 75th centile from surveys
    E. the dose from an examination must only be within the set diagnostic reference level

Q 16. During fluoroscopy:

    A. effective dose is best estimated using a dose area product meter
    B. a dose area product meter is attached beneath the patient when using over couch screening
    C. effective dose can be measured directly
    D. male gonad dose can be estimated by attaching a thermoluminescent dosimeter to the scrotum
    E. the Health and Safety Executive must be informed if the actual exposure is twice the intended

Examination Six

Questions

Q 17. **Film γ depends on:**

A. kV
B. filtration
C. development time
D. fixation
E. use of intensifying screen

Q 18. **Screen unsharpness is affected by:**

A. type of film used
B. thickness of screen
C. density of screen
D. X-ray energy
E. amount of backscatter from the patient

Q 19. **Regarding the image intensifier:**

A. the input screen is made of calcium tungstate
B. photocathode converts X-rays to light
C. spatial resolution of the largest field is greater than the smallest
D. the overall brightness gain is 10,000
E. diameter of output phosphor is 2.5 cm

Q 20. **In a γ camera:**

A. different thickness crystals can be fitted to a γ camera to carry out imaging with different nuclides
B. non-uniformity is caused more by the scintillator crystal than by the photomultiplier tubes
C. the magnitude of the light pulse is proportional to the energy absorbed in the crystal
D. the pulse height analysers window width determines the sensitivity of the system
E. collimators are primarily used to absorb scattered radiation

Q 21. Technetium-99m:

A. has a photon energy of 0.12 MeV

B. has a radioactive daughter product

C. is an example of electron capture decay

D. is a daughter product of the parent nuclide ^{131}I

E. is a generator produced radionuclide

Q 22. In nuclear medicine:

A. the ideal radionuclide is a pure γ emitter

B. lead aprons should be used if γ-ray energies are greater than 140 keV

C. all radioactive waste must be disposed off by a specialist waste contractor

D. radioactive injections should not be given to pregnant patients

E. while the patient is in a scanning room, it must always be designated at least a supervised area

Q 23. Regarding quality assessment of X-ray equipment:

A. image uniformity in CT is measured with a water phantom

B. focal spot size can be measured with a star pattern

C. test objects can be used to measure low contrast detection in fluoroscopy

D. exposure time can be measured with an ion chamber and electrometer

E. maximum tube potential cannot be measured by penetrameter

Q 24. In computed tomography:

   A. the Hounsfield unit value for fat is approximately −200

   B. a displayed pixel value is related to linear attenuation coefficient μ

   C. the photoelectric effect predominates

   D. axial resolution decreases with increasing slice width

   E. a narrow selected window width improves displayed image contrast

Q 25. In computed tomography scanning:

   A. collimation is done solely to decrease scatter

   B. low power X-ray sources are used to lower the dose to the patient

   C. X-ray tubes where the anode rotates faster, are used in spiral scanning compared to axial scanning

   D. use the results from Fourier transforms to reconstruct the image

   E. a bow tie filter is used

Q 1. **The range of a charged particle in a medium:**

- **A.** is proportional to the initial energy of the particle
- **B.** is independent of the mass of the particle
- **C.** increases as the velocity of the charged particle increases
- **D.** increases as the charge of the particle decreases
- **E.** is independent of the density of the medium

Q 2. **Compton collisions:**

- **A.** occur when a photon interacts with a nucleus
- **B.** produce photoelectrons and scattered photons
- **C.** cause ionisation of atoms
- **D.** mainly occur when low energy photons interact with high atomic number materials
- **E.** result in partial absorption

Q 3. **Scattered photons produced by the Compton interaction:**

- **A.** have a higher energy if scattered in the forward direction
- **B.** have an intensity greater than that of the primary beam
- **C.** produce ionisation
- **D.** result from the interaction with free electrons
- **E.** are the same as the recoil electron

Q 4. Characteristic radiation:

A. is characteristic of the tube voltage used
B. has an energy related to the filament temperature
C. is only produced when a specific voltage waveform is employed
D. is characteristic of the target material
F. its energy increases as the atomic number of the target material increases

Q 5. The inherent filtration of a diagnostic X-ray tube:

A. is mainly due to oil
B. is normally equivalent to 2 mm of aluminium
C. depends on the kV across the tube
D. is responsible for absorbing short wavelength X-rays
E. is responsible for absorbing high energy X-rays

Q 6. The binding energy of an electron is:

A. its kinetic energy
B. greater for an electron in an M-orbit than for one in an L-orbit
C. the energy required to remove the electron from an orbit
D. normally measured in volts
E. dependent on the atomic number of the element

Q 7. In the interaction of an electron stream with the target in an X-ray tube:

A. the target is positive relative to the cathode
B. tungsten is suitable target material
C. in the bremmstrahlung phenomenon an Auger electron is produced
D. in the bremmstrahlung phenomenon the maximum wavelength of the X-ray photon produced will depend on the kVp
E. rotation of the target increases the effective focal spot

Q 8. **The quality of an X-ray beam depends directly on:**

A. the peak voltage applied to the tube
B. the waveform of the voltage applied to the tube
C. the tube current
D. total filtration of the beam
E. atomic number of the target

Q 9. **Exponential X-ray attenuation:**

A. depends on the inverse square law
B. if a 1 mm thickness decreases the beam intensity by a factor of 2 then 1 cm will decrease the beam intensity by a factor of 20
C. applies to the normal X-ray spectrum but not to a mono-energetic beam
D. does not decrease the beam intensity to zero
E. the linear attenuation coefficient is proportional to the half value layer

Q 10. **Concerning isotopes:**

A. the effective half-life is always less than the biological half-life or the physical half-life
B. metastable isotopes usually decay by γ emission
C. α emission results in the mass number decreasing by two
D. with β emission the mass number changes
E. α emission is easily stopped by paper

Examination Seven

Questions

Q 11. Regarding the effects of ionising radiation:

A. descendents of patients undergoing radiotherapy have been shown to have an increased incidence of congenital defects

B. cataract formation is an example of a deterministic (non-stochastic) effect

C. the probability of stochastic effects occurring do not increase with increased dose

D. irradiation of the fetus at 6 weeks after conception carries a higher risk of organ malformation than irradiation of the fetus at 10 weeks after conception

E. the effective (whole-body) dose of a radiological procedure is calculated by adding the doses applied to each organ by the procedure

Q 12. A thermoluminescent detector such as lithium fluoride:

A. has a linear response to dose over a very wide dose range

B. can be used to measure both dose and dose rate

C. can differentiate the energy of radiation

D. can be used for patient and personal dose monitoring

E. has an accuracy better than 5%

Q 13. Which of the following are true regarding dosimetry units?

A. the absorbed dose to an organ depends on its mass

B. the radiation weighting factor W_R applies to low doses and dose rates

C. the unit of equivalent dose is the Sievert

D. the unit of effective dose is the Sievert

E. absorbed dose and equivalent dose are numerically equal for X-rays

Q 14. The Ionising Radiation Regulations (1999):

A. state that there should not be any measurable radiation exceeding background radiation on the outside of the shielding of equipment containing radioactive substance

B. do not apply to radiation beam therapy

C. state that nursing mothers should not be employed in work involving a high risk of radioactive contamination

D. state that an investigation should be held when any employee incurs a dose of more than three-tenths of the annual dose limit

E. state that it is not permissible to allow trainees of less than 18 years into controlled areas

Q 15. Concerning radiation protection:

A. equivalent doses allow a range of non-uniform organ doses to be combined as a single number

B. the radiation weighting factor is the same for α particles and γ-rays

C. X-rays have a radiation weighting factor of one

D. absorbed dose and equivalent dose are numerically equivalent for diagnostic range X-rays

E. α particles have a similar radiation weighting factor to high energy neutrons

Q 16. Under IRR (1999), the following dose limits are correct:

A. 20 mSv effective dose per year (in certain circumstances 100 mSv over 5 years)

B. 150 mSv to the lens of the eye of a trainee under 18

C. equivalent dose of 20 mSv per annum

D. effective dose of 15 mSv to a member of the public

E. equivalent dose to abdomen of 13 mSv per trimester to pregnant women

Q 17. Regarding the practice of radiation protection:

A. a worker cannot be classified on the basis of their hand exposure alone

B. a beam directed at the floor has a lower weighting factor than a beam directed at the ceiling in determining the thickness of shielding

C. a brick wall would provide better shielding than 10 cm concrete in the diagnostic range (all other things being equal)

D. workers are not legally required to be individually monitored

E. doses would be expected to be higher in a controlled area than in a supervised area

Q 18. The characteristic curve of a film-screen system:

A. is derived by exposing the system to a series of exposures

B. is a plot of the log of the optical density against the log relative exposure

C. the base density is greater in tinted films

D. the average gradient of the curve is independent of the grain size

E. as the curve moves to the right the sensitivity increases

Q 19. In the films used in radiography:

A. the emulsion crystals contains more iodide than bromide

B. the latent image is produced at the sensitivity specks

C. the screen coating the posterior emulsion functions by absorbing light produced by the anterior emulsion

D. the agent in the development process that produces the silver metallic grains from the latent image should be an electron donor

E. increasing the developer temperature would be expected to increase the speed of the film

Q 20. Subject contrast is generally decreased by:

  A. film fog
  B. tissues with similar densities
  C. using 30 kVp instead of 60 kVp in mammography
  D. the use of contrast media
  E. using a lower total exposure (mAs)

Q 21. The following are true of the image intensifier:

  A. the input phosphor is usually made of zinc-cadmium sulphide
  B. light is produced at both the input and output phosphor
  C. the area of the input phosphor is larger than the area of the output phosphor
  D. the periphery of the final image is brighter than the centre of the image
  E. magnification is normally achieved by reducing the distance between the input and output phosphors

Q 22. In the γ camera:

  A. the choice of a collimator is influenced by the size of the organ to be imaged
  B. increasing the thickness of the crystal increases its intrinsic resolution
  C. the pulse height selector discriminates between different amounts of pulses received by the crystal
  D. each point of light in the crystal results in an output from more than one photomultiplier tube
  E. variation in the image of a uniform source is caused mainly by variations in the thickness of the NaI (Tl) crystal

Q 23. The effective dose to a patient in nuclear medicine:

    A. depends on the choice of radiopharmaceutical
    B. is independent of the physical half-life of the radionuclide
    C. will be reduced if a lower energy γ emitter is used
    D. is less than 10 mSv for the majority of common diagnostic studies
    E. can be estimated if the residence times in individual organs are known

Q 24. In computed tomography imaging:

    A. the partial volume effect is when the cross sectional area of the patient exceeds the internal size of the scanner
    B. beam hardening corrections may be aided by a bow-tie filter
    C. contrast which arises from the attenuated beam is due to photoelectric interactions
    D. uses low power X-ray sources to lower the dose to the patient
    E. have more than one X-ray source if they are capable of spiral scanning

Q 25. The following are true of image quality in CT:

    A. using a narrower window reduces the effect of noise
    B. increasing the slice thickness increases the effect of noise
    C. line-pair resolution is generally better than that obtainable in film-screen radiography
    D. the phenomenon called 'cupping' (abnormally lower attenuation at the centre of the CT image) is usually caused by detector malfunction
    E. in a scan using helical (spiral) scanning resolution is improved by increasing the pitch

Section 2 – Answers

A 1.   **A.** true   **B.** true   **C.** true   **D.** false   **E.** true

Beta decay results in the emission of an electron from the nucleus. This may be a positive or negative electron. Beta particles are light charged particles, having a charge of e, are ionising and are typically stopped by a millimetre of aluminium.

In β− decay the atomic number increases by one and the mass number remains constant.

In β+ decay the atomic number decreases by one and the mass number remains constant.

A 2.   **A.** true   **B.** true   **C.** false   **D.** true   **E.** true

Electron capture occurs in neutron poor radionuclides. In the nucleus the captured electron combines with a proton to form a neutron. The vacancy in the electron shell is filled by an outer orbital electron and the difference in energy between the orbits results in the emission of characteristic X-rays.

Example: Iodine-125 and Iodine-123.

The atomic number is decreased by one and the atomic mass number remains constant.

A 3.   **A.** true   **B.** false   **C.** false   **D.** true   **E.** false

Isotopes of an element are nuclides that have the same number of protons, i.e. identical atomic numbers, the same position in the periodic table, and chemical and metabolic properties.

They have a different number of neutrons, a different mass number and therefore density and different physical properties.

A 4. **A.** true **B.** false **C.** true **D.** true **E.** false

Unstable nuclides, which have a neutron excess or deficit, are radioactive and decay through a decay series until they become stable by emitting α, β or γ radiation.

The activity of a radionuclide is the number of decays per second. The unit of activity is the Becquerel (Bq).

The daughter product is not always radioactive, i.e. it may be the stable nuclide at the end of the decay series.

A 5. **A.** true **B.** true **C.** true **D.** false **E.** true

$$\text{Photon energy (keV)} = \frac{1.24}{\text{wavelength (in nm)}}$$

$$E \text{ (photon energy)} = h \text{ (Planck's constant)} \times f \text{ (frequency)}$$

The half value layer (HVL) is a measure of the penetrating power and the effective energy of the beam. The HVL and effective energy of an X-ray beam increases as the applied kV is increased.

The heel effect is independent of keV and results in a relative decrease in X-ray intensity on the anode side of the beam.

A 6. **A.** false **B.** true **C.** false **D.** false **E.** true

The photoelectric effect is the interaction of a photon and a bound electron and occurs approximately 10–30% of the time for a typical diagnostic spectrum in soft tissue. Interaction occurs with the K-shell electron about 80% of the time and the L-shell electron about 20% of the time.

The photoelectric interaction coefficient τ is proportional to $\rho Z^3/E^3$, where ρ is the physical density; Z is the atomic number and E is the photon energy.

Therefore as the photon energy increases the photoelectric interaction occurs less frequently. It does result in the emission of characteristic X-rays from the atom but these are low energy in low Z materials and are absorbed locally.

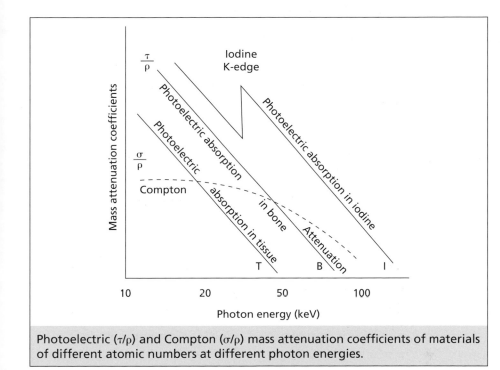

Photoelectric (τ/ρ) and Compton (σ/ρ) mass attenuation coefficients of materials of different atomic numbers at different photon energies.

A 7.   A. false   B. false   C. true   D. true   E. true

In the Compton process a photon interacts with a free electron which recoils taking away some of the energy of the photon as kinetic energy. The photon is scattered in a new direction, with reduced energy. Scatter of photons can be in all directions.

At 30 keV in soft tissues 50% of attenuation will be due to the Compton effect and 50% due to photoelectric interaction. At 50 keV in bone 50% of attenuation will be due to the Compton effect and 50% due to the photoelectric effect.

The probability that the Compton process will occur is proportional to physical density and electron density. It is independent of the atomic number of the material as the number of electrons per unit mass is approximately constant for most materials (where Z/A is approximately 0.5) with the exception of hydrogen (where Z/A = 1).

σ is proportional to ρ/E and is independent of Z, where σ is the probability that the Compton process will occur.

A 8.   **A.** false   **B.** true   **C.** true   **D.** false   **E.** false

The rotating anode tube consists of:

- An anode disk, 7–10 cm or more in diameter, usually made of tungsten-rhenium alloy. This material has better thermal characteristics than pure tungsten and does not roughen with use as quickly.
- A thin molybdenum stem
- A blackened copper rotor, this increases radiation heat
- Bearings, lubricated with a soft metal such as silver, which enables the rotor to rotate around the axle

The molybdenum stem is sufficiently long and narrow to control the amount of heat that is conducted to the rotor, so that it is not in danger of overheating and seizing up.

A 9.   **A.** false   **B.** true   **C.** false   **D.** false   **E.** true

The quality (intensity plotted as a function of photon energy) of the beam from an X-ray tube depends on:

- Peak tube potential (kVp) since a higher kVp produces a beam of higher average energy
- Rectification of the tube voltage, since this determines the kV variation with time
- Filtration, since a filter is used to harden the beam (remove a greater proportion of lower energy photons)

The tube current (mA) does not alter the quality.

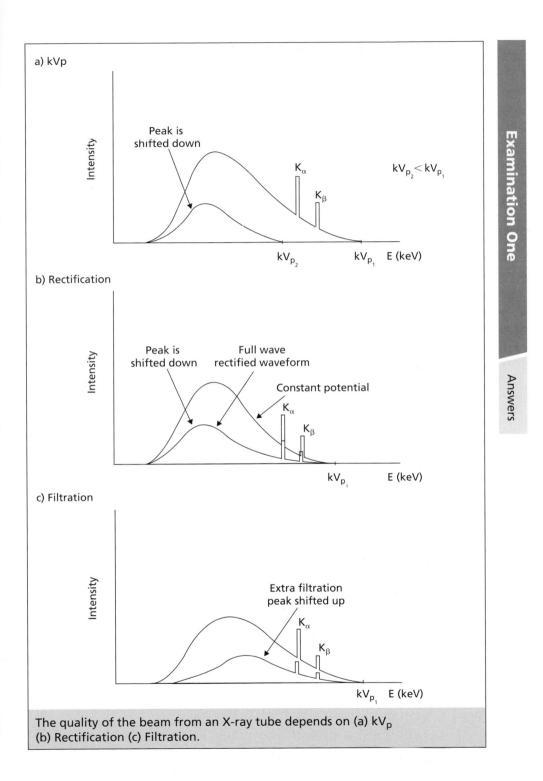

a) kVp

Intensity

Peak is
shifted down

K_α

K_β

$kV_{p_2} < kV_{p_1}$

kV_{p_2} kV_{p_1} E (keV)

b) Rectification

Intensity

Peak is
shifted down

Full wave
rectified waveform

Constant potential

K_α

K_β

kV_{p_1} E (keV)

c) Filtration

Intensity

Extra filtration
peak shifted up

K_α

K_β

kV_{p_1} E (keV)

The quality of the beam from an X-ray tube depends on (a) kV_p
(b) Rectification (c) Filtration.

A **10.** **A.** true **B.** true **C.** true **D.** false **E.** false

Scatter reaching the film may be reduced by:

- air gap
- use of a grid
- use of a cone by reducing the field size
- compression of patient
- lower kV

A **11.** **A.** false **B.** true **C.** false **D.** false **E.** false

The maximum energy in the X-ray spectrum is determined by the peak tube potential (kVp) across the X-ray tube.

Low energies (18–20 keV) are required in order to distinguish the soft tissues by photoelectric interaction.

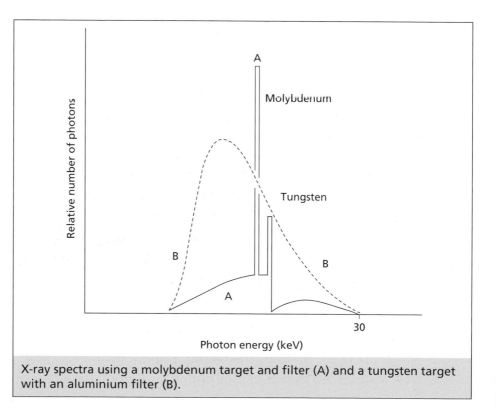

X-ray spectra using a molybdenum target and filter (A) and a tungsten target with an aluminium filter (B).

The target material used is molybdenum. It produces characteristic radiation of 17.9 keV and 19.5 keV.

A K-edge beam filter of molybdenum is used to reduce all other energy X-rays in the spectrum as the filter is relatively transparent to its own characteristic (K-edge) radiation.

Typical glandular breast dose from a single film is less than 2 mGy.

A focus to film distance of approximately 60 cm is used.

A **12.** **A.** true   **B.** true   **C.** false   **D.** true   **E.** false

Deterministic effects are due to radiation induced cell death. The cell population might recover.

They do not occur below a threshold dose.

The severity of effect increases with dose.

Examples are erythema, hair loss, eye cataracts, and sterilisation.

A **13.** **A.** true   **B.** true   **C.** true   **D.** true   **E.** true

A Radiation Protection Adviser (RPA) is responsible for advising the employer on the application of IRR (1999). They must be consulted over all new installations and on the designation of areas. A Radiation Protection Supervisor (RPS) must be appointed in all areas where there are local rules, whether controlled or supervised areas.

Classified workers are employees likely to receive an effective dose greater than 6 mSv or greater than 3/10 of an employee equivalent dose limit, e.g. for lens of the eye or skin.

A **14.** **A.** false   **B.** true   **C.** false   **D.** false   **E.** true

It is the responsibility of the employer under quality assurance to monitor and maintain the safety of equipment.

A controlled area is one in which doses are likely to exceed 30% of a dose limit per annum. A supervised area is one in which doses are likely to exceed 10% of an equivalent dose limit, or exceed a whole body effective dose of 1 mSv per year.

These areas are defined in the local rules.

Systems of work are procedures to keep dose as low as reasonably practicable (ALARP) and <30% of dose limits.

A **15.** **A.** false **B.** true **C.** true **D.** false **E.** false

Doses must be kept as low as reasonably practicable.

Practitioners and operators shall have successfully completed training, including theoretical knowledge and practical experience.

An ARSAC license is granted to an individual practitioner.

All NHS hospitals are subject to IRR (1999), IRMER (2000) and RSA (1993).

A **16.** **A.** false **B.** false **C.** false **D.** false **E.** true

Workers who receive less than 30% can be classified. If they receive more, they must be classified.

It is unusual for any X-ray department worker to be classified.

Records must be kept for 50 years.

A **17.** **A.** true **B.** false **C.** true **D.** false **E.** false

The current statutory dose limit for members of the public is 1 mSv per annum. In comparison the natural background radiation dose is around 2.2 mSv per annum in the south east of the UK.

The effective dose from an AP pelvis radiograph is approximately 0.7 mSv.

A member of staff must become a classified worker when their whole body dose is likely to exceed 6 mSv per annum, or if they are likely to exceed 3/10 of any other equivalent dose limit.

The lifetime risk of harm is approximately 1 in 14,000 per mSv (so, for 2 mSv the risk would be approximately 1 in 7,000).

A 18. **A.** false   **B.** true   **C.** true   **D.** true   **E.** false

The film characteristic curve is a plot of optical density versus log of exposure.

Gamma can be defined as the average slope between two points on the characteristic curve, normally 0.25 and 2.0. Sometimes γ can be specified at one point on the curve to reflect the slope of the curve at a particular density.

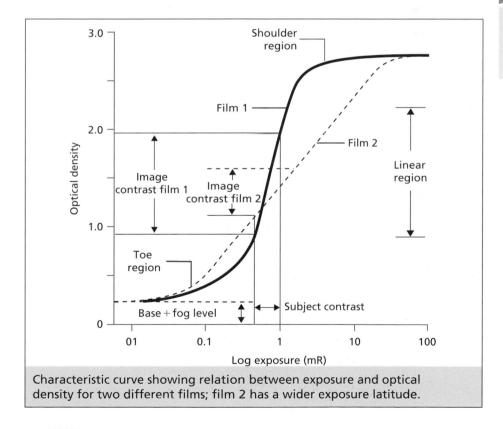

Characteristic curve showing relation between exposure and optical density for two different films; film 2 has a wider exposure latitude.

If $\gamma > 1$ there will be an increase in radiographic contrast.

An increase in grain size is associated with increased speed and a small increase in γ.

A uniform grain size increases film γ, whereas a large range reduces film γ.

A 19. **A.** true **B.** false **C.** true **D.** false **E.** true

Radiographic contrast = film contrast $\times$ subject contrast

Radiographic contrast is the density difference between two defined areas in a radiographic image.

Film contrast is a function of the film screen combination.

It is affected by the characteristic curve, film density and processing, as well as by the use or not of screens. Use of screens can increase the γ when compared to a system without screens.

A 20. **A.** false **B.** false **C.** false **D.** true **E.** true

Subject contrast is formed as a result of the range of the radiation intensities transmitted by the patient.

It is altered by:

- kVp
- density
- thickness
- Z
- scatter
- the use of a contrast agent

A 21. **A.** true **B.** true **C.** true **D.** true **E.** false

The effective dose for a PET ^{18}F-FDG scan is 5 mSv. The annual dose limit for members of the public is 1 mSv. Natural background radiation averages about 2.2 mSv in the south-east of the UK. The average annual dose for diagnostic medical radiation is 0.37 mSv. The entrance surface dose of a chest radiograph is 0.3 mGy.

A 22. A. true   **B.** true   **C.** false   **D.** false   **E.** false

A Huttner line pair phantom, part of the Leeds test object kit, may be used to measure limiting resolution from the monitor image. During fluoroscopy the input dose rate is normally between 0.2 and 2 μGys^{-1} at the image intensifier input plane. The input phosphor consists of caesium iodide. The output phosphor is formed from zinc-cadmium-sulphide (silver doped).

$$\text{Brightness gain} = \text{flux gain} \times \text{minification gain}$$

The smaller the field of view selected, the more magnified the image appears, so improving the limiting spatial resolution detected.

A 23. A. true   **B.** false   **C.** true   **D.** true   **E.** false

The TV system limits the spatial resolution due to:

- The mosaic structure of the TV camera image plate
- Line structure of the TV image which affects vertical resolution
- Band width of the TV monitor electronics which affects horizontal resolution

The resolution of a TV screen is 1 lp/mm (line pairs per mm). The resolution of a film/screen combination is 5–20 lp/mm.

Film averaging can reduce quantum noise. Noise is random so averaging frames will reduce noise. As a result the signal noise ratio is improved by a factor equal to the square root of the number of frames averaged. Focus skin distances must not be less than 30 cm and should preferably be greater than 45 cm, especially on non-mobile X-ray systems.

A dose area product (DAP) meter is mounted on the diaphragm housing, close to the tube focus and away from the patient to avoid radiation back scattered from the patient. It can be readily used to estimate the energy imparted to the patient in an examination.

A 24. A. false **B.** false **C.** true **D.** true **E.** true

A pure γ emitter is ideal, i.e. a radiopharmaceutical which decays by isomeric transition or electron capture, as producing extra particles only increases patient dose.

A short half-life will minimise irradiation of the patient and stability in vivo enhances imaging.

Radiopharmaceuticals with a high mass number are more likely to decay by α or β emission. Ideally the daughter product will be stable, leading to minimal further irradiation of the patient.

A 25. A. true **B.** true **C.** true **D.** false **E.** false

In a 4th generation scanner the detectors are stationary, only the X-ray tube rotates whereas in 3rd generation scanners both the detector array and tube rotate.

Spatial resolution deteriorates with increased slice width or increased pixel size.

The tube anode/cathode axis is perpendicular to the fan beam plane and parallel to the detector array.

Increasing slice thickness will increase the partial volume effect.

Question	A	B	C	D	E
1	T	T	T	F	T
2	T	T	F	T	T
3	T	F	F	T	F
4	T	F	T	T	F
5	T	T	T	F	T
6	F	T	F	F	T
7	F	F	T	T	T
8	F	T	T	F	F
9	F	T	F	F	T
10	T	T	T	F	F
11	F	T	F	F	F
12	T	T	F	T	F
13	T	T	T	T	T
14	F	T	F	F	T
15	F	T	T	F	F
16	F	F	F	F	T
17	T	F	T	F	F
18	F	T	T	T	F
19	T	F	T	F	T
20	F	F	F	T	T
21	T	T	T	T	F
22	T	T	F	F	F
23	T	F	T	T	F
24	F	F	T	T	T
25	T	T	T	F	F

Examination One

Answers

A 1.   **A.** true   **B.** true   **C.** false   **D.** false   **E.** true

β− decay occurs in neutron rich nuclides. A neutron is transformed into a proton and electron and the electron is emitted from the nucleus with a range of kinetic energies up to a maximum value. The atomic number is increased by one and the atomic mass remains constant.

β+ decay occurs in neutron poor nuclides. A proton is transformed into a neutron and a positive electron (an anti-electron positron) and the positron is emitted from the nucleus. The atomic number is decreased by one and the atomic mass remains constant.

The electron charge is denoted by e and is of opposite sign for electrons and positrons, the electrons being negative. As the particles have kinetic energy they will cause ionisation as they have collisions and lose energy along their tracks in a medium.

A 2.   **A.** false   **B.** true   **C.** false   **D.** false   **E.** false

The nucleus contains neutrons and protons, except hydrogen which only contains a proton.

A 3.   **A.** false   **B.** true   **C.** true   **D.** true   **E.** false

The law of radioactive decay states that the activity of a radioactive sample decreases by equal fractions (percentages) in equal intervals of time. The rate of decay of a given sample (number of nuclei undergoing a radioactive transition per unit time) is proportional to the number of remaining nuclei present at that time.

The effective half-life is a result of two contributory processes. Firstly the elimination from the body of a radionuclide with a given biological half-life (t_{biol}) and the physical decay half-life (t_{phys}) of the nuclide. As both processes act to reduce the amount of radionuclide present the effective half-life (t_{eff}) is always shorter than either the physical or biological half-life. The quantities are related as follows:

$$\frac{1}{t_{eff}} = \frac{1}{t_{biol}} + \frac{1}{t_{phys}}$$

There may be several γ-rays emitted during a radioactive decay of a given radionuclide. These have a few specific energies, which form a line spectrum, that is characteristic of the nuclide which emits them.

Temperature will not affect nuclear decay processes.

A 4. **A.** false **B.** true **C.** false **D.** true **E.** false

The photoelectric effect is the interaction of a photon and a bound electron that is ejected from the atom. The atom is then ionised.

The photoelectric attenuation coefficient is proportional to Z^3/E^3 where E is the photon energy and predominates for contrast media, lead and the materials used in films and screens because of their higher atomic number than tissue. It also gives rise to contrast between bone and soft tissue because of the higher atomic number for bone than soft tissue and so is important in diagnostic radiology.

A 5. **A.** false **B.** true **C.** false **D.** false **E.** false

In the Compton process a photon interacts with a free electron. Greater the angle of scatter of the photon greater is the energy and range of the recoil electron and greater the loss of energy of the incident photon.

The probability of the Compton process depends on physical density (mass per unit volume) × number of electrons per unit mass.

The Compton process is the predominant process for air, water and soft tissues at photon energies above approximately 30 keV.

A 6. **A.** true   **B.** true   **C.** false   **D.** true   **E.** false

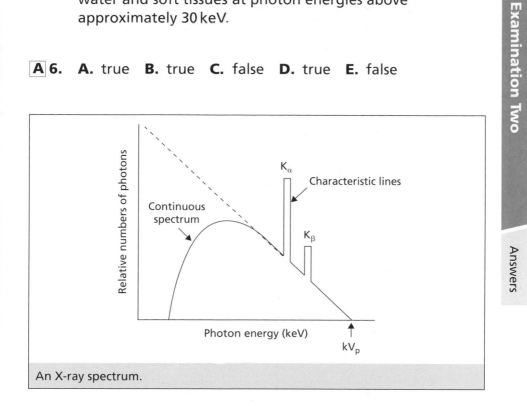

An X-ray spectrum.

The peak tube potential gives the maximum energy that an electron can have to collide with the anode, and hence the maximum X-ray photon energy possible in the beam. The X-ray yield or efficiency of X-ray production increases with atomic number of the target anode.

The characteristic lines in the spectrum are characteristic of the target material. Filtration tends to reduce intensity and also affect the spectral shape. The spectrum is independent of the distance from anode to cathode (the voltage difference is the same) and the tube current merely changes the number of photons, not the spectral shape.

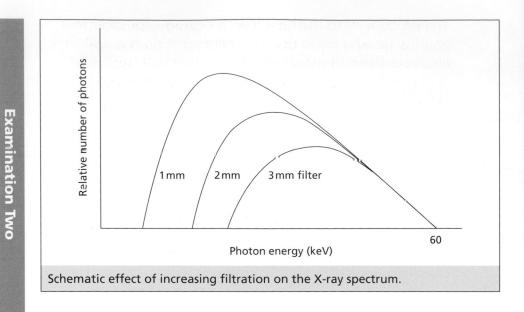

1 mm   2 mm   3 mm filter

Relative number of photons

Photon energy (keV)

60

Schematic effect of increasing filtration on the X-ray spectrum.

A 7.   **A.** false   **B.** true   **C.** true   **D.** true   **E.** false

With a rectified or non-rectified single phase generator there is a different distribution of X-ray energies at different times as the tube potential varies over the mains cycle from maximum to minimum.

With three phase or constant potential kV waveforms the tube potential is close to the peak tube potential over the whole mains cycle so on average the voltage is greater and certainly closer to the set kVp than for a single phase generator. Hence for a single phase generator there is a larger proportion of lower energy photons compared to a constant phase generator for a given maximum tube potential (kVp).

The lower mean energy of the single phase spectrum means that the beam is less penetrating and a higher entrance surface dose (ESD) must be given to the patient in order to expose the image receptor to the required dose. Overall a greater X-ray dose to the patient results.

For given values of kVp and mA the three phase generator generates more X-ray photons and hence a greater tube output. This allows a shorter exposure time to attain the required receptor dose. One does not always require a three phase generator to use a high speed tube, in practice high speed tubes tend to have three phase generators however.

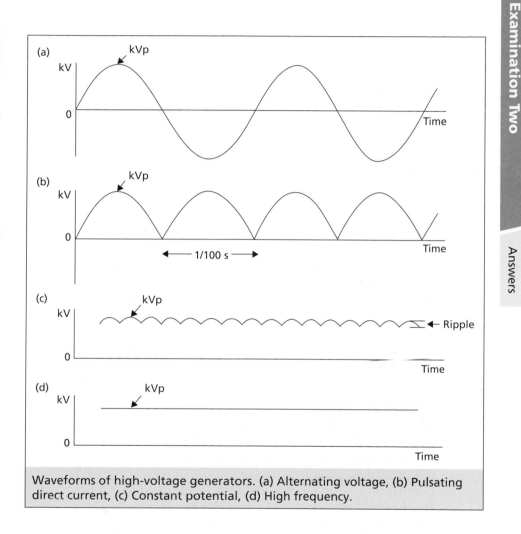

Waveforms of high-voltage generators. (a) Alternating voltage, (b) Pulsating direct current, (c) Constant potential, (d) High frequency.

A 8. **A.** true **B.** true **C.** true **D.** false **E.** false

The output is proportional to Z, kV², mA, and 1/d²
(where d = distance from target).

The output increases with a constant potential compared
to a single phase waveform. The output decreases with
increasing filtration.

A 9. **A.** false **B.** false **C.** true **D.** false **E.** true

X-rays are produced when fast moving electrons are
suddenly stopped by impact on a metal target. The
electrons penetrate several micrometers into the target
and lose their energy in two ways:

- Interaction with the outer electrons of the atoms
  producing heat (99%)
- Interaction with either the inner shells of the atoms,
  or the field of the nucleus (bremsstrahlung interaction)
  producing X-rays (1%)

A 10. **A.** true **B.** true **C.** true **D.** true **E.** false

Compression moves overlying tissues laterally, reduces the
thickness of irradiated tissue and so decreases scatter and
improves contrast.

Film latitude refers to the range in optical densities that
can be visualised. In mammography the atomic number
does not differ very much between tissues therefore the
range can afford to be small. A greater film screen γ is
preferable as this gives greater radiographic contrast.
Contraindications to compression are intolerance and the
presence of an open skin wound.

A 11. **A.** false **B.** false **C.** true **D.** true **E.** false

There is a threshold below which there is no effect.

The threshold dose varies for different pathological
conditions.

Pathology	Threshold dose (Gy)
Prodromal syndrome	0.5
Erythema	2.0
Hair loss	3.0
Cataracts	2–5
Temporary suppression of ovulation	1.5–5
Temporary loss of sperm	0.3–2
Death (whole body dose)	5 (LD_{50})

Once above the deterministic threshold the severity of effect is related to dose. The probability of effects occurring depends linearly on dose with stochastic effects. Above a threshold dose, deterministic effects will be demonstrated.

A 12. **A.** false **B.** false **C.** true **D.** false **E.** false

Using a higher kV increases the tube output per mAs and makes the beam more penetrating, and increases the proportion of photons incident on the patient actually reaching the image receptor. As a result, a lower entrance skin dose is needed for the same exit dose (and hence receptor dose). Therefore increasing the kV reduces the skin dose and the dose to the deeper tissues. This phenomenon is most pronounced for tissues near the surface and has little effect for doses near the exit site of the beam.

Optical density is controlled by kV ($\propto kV^4$).

The object of filtration is to remove a large proportion of the lower energy photons before they reach the skin or deeper. It reduces the overall intensity of the beam however so the mAs may need to be increased but the overall effect is to reduce entrance surface dose.

Smaller field sizes save dose because they reduce the size of the irradiated anatomy and scatter. The percentage depth dose (100% being the entrance surface dose) tends to be greater with larger field sizes at a given depth.

A larger focal spot has no effect on dose (for a given target angle).

A 13. A. true   **B.** false   **C.** true   **D.** false   **E.** false

Dose investigation levels are set within a department and are investigated if exceeded. The investigation level would certainly be set below the 3/10 of a maximum annual dose limit.

A classified worker is an employee likely to receive greater than 6 mSv effective dose or greater than 3/10 of any other employee equivalent dose limit (e.g. skin, extremities). In this case the employee should be classified as they have already reached 30% of the whole body effective dose limit. Classified workers require a yearly medical by an appointed doctor to be certified fit. In this case the medical would be as a result of the process of classification and not because of the 6 mSv dose received. The worker does not have to stop radiation work but changes may be made to their working practices as a result of the local investigation into the dose received to ensure doses are being kept as low as reasonably practicable.

The Health and Safety Executive should be notified of the following:

- dose exceeding dose limit
- medical exposure much greater than intended
- loss or theft of source
- release or spillage leading to significant contamination

A 14. **A.** false   **B.** true   **C.** false   **D.** false   **E.** true

The RPA normally works in the medical physics department. The radiation protection committee should have management representation.

The General Practitioner (GP) is the referrer and is not a practitioner or operator under the IRMER Regulations. The radiographer is an operator under IRMER (2000) and normally would not be acting as a practitioner under IRMER in this context.

Authorisation can be performed by the practitioner or by an operator acting under written guidelines.

A 15. **A.** false   **B.** true   **C.** false   **D.** true   **E.** false

Physical direction of an examination may be performed by other staff identified and instructed by the ARSAC certificate holder. The application is signed by the radiopharmacist, senior scientist responsible for the facilities and the RPA.

An individual granted an ARSAC certificate has to renew it every 5 years. Research ARSAC licences may be for a shorter fixed period or number of patients. The ARSAC licence holder is ultimately responsible for the discharge of patients. The maximum dose to the patient is defined in the ARSAC certificate by the maximum activity of the radiopharmaceutical that can be administered.

A 16. **A.** true   **B.** false   **C.** false   **D.** false   **E.** true

Most health workers would probably receive less than 1 mSv per annum. Doses to staff groups vary but a significant amount of fluoroscopy or interventional radiology could mean greater doses for those staff. In many cases cardiologists get greater doses than radiologists who in turn receive more than radiographers.

IRMER (2000) requires diagnostic reference levels (DRLs) to be set for investigations. There are no dose limits for patients undergoing medical exposures under IRR (1999). IRR (1999) sets dose limits for workers and members of the public, of whom patients while in the waiting room are regarded as members of the public.

A 17. A. false **B.** false **C.** false **D.** true **E.** true

A diagnostic reference level is a dose level, or amount of radioactivity used in a diagnostic procedure for typical examinations. It is not a dose limit.

Each hospital sets its own DRL for a given examination and piece of equipment on which the examination is carried out. These DRLs should be compared with the national or European reference dose levels where these are available. DRLs can be assessed using entrance surface dose (ESD), kV and mAs, dose area product (DAP) or screening time.

Different DRLs are set for different age ranges in paediatrics.

DRLs should not normally be exceeded under standard conditions.

A 18. A. false **B.** true **C.** false **D.** true **E.** true

The DAP meter ionisation chamber is mounted on the light beam diaphragm, well away from the patient to avoid back scatter.

The ESD for a lateral lumbar spine is approximately 10 mGy.

The ESD for an AP abdomen is approximately 4 mGy.

The time of onset for a transient erythema is between 2 and 24 h and 2 Gy is the lower threshold dose.

A 19. **A.** false   **B.** true   **C.** true   **D.** true   **E.** false

Intensifying screens have the following advantages:

- Patient dose reduction
- Shorter exposure times, so reducing motion artefact
- Improves image contrast
- But reduce spatial resolution

Screen speed can be increased by increasing:

- Thickness of the phosphor layer
- Crystal size
- Conversion efficiency
- Absorption efficiency

Intensifying screens increase γ from about 2 to 3.

A 20. **A.** false   **B.** false   **C.** false   **D.** true   **E.** true

Sharpness or blurring is the ability of X-ray film/film-screen combination to reproduce a distinct edge as a line. In the image receptor the thickness of the screen affects the diffusion of light out from where the X-ray photon is absorbed and hence the resolution. Resolution is also affected by crossover of light from front to rear emulsions and vice versa, grain size, beam parallax and screen film contact. Image sharpness is also affected by patient motion, geometry (penumbra, magnification and focal spot size).

A 21. **A.** true   **B.** true   **C.** false   **D.** false   **E.** false

$$\text{Brightness gain} = \text{flux gain} \times \text{minification gain}$$

$$\text{Flux gain} = \text{acceleration of electrons by potential applied across image intensifier}$$

$$\text{Minification gain} = \frac{(\text{diameter input phosphor})^2}{(\text{diameter output phosphor})^2}$$

A 22. A. false **B.** false **C.** false **D.** true **E.** false

The Zn-Cd-sulphide output screen converts the electron beam (not X-rays) back into green light. The camera pick up tube may have a lag of several hundred milliseconds thus causing image lag. However in comparison the lag of the image intensifier tube is negligible being around only 1 ms.

Intensification factor = minification gain × flux gain
(up to 15,000 for large image intensifiers)

A 23. A. false **B.** false **C.** true **D.** true **E.** false

kV can be measured directly using a potential divider or indirectly with a penetrameter. The actual kV should be within ±5%.

An ion chamber measures dose, not time. A spinning lead top on top of a film during an exposure can be used to measure exposure time. On modern equipment, this function has been added to the kV meter to produce a dual purpose device.

Fluoroscopy with an image intensifier-TV achieves spatial resolution of 1 lp/mm. Total filtration should be 2.5 mm Al except for mammography and some dental units and this will generally be satisfied for a measured beam HVL of 2.8 mm Al at 80 kVp.

Film-screen contact can be checked by radiography of a perforated metal sheet placed on top of the cassette.

A 24. A. true **B.** false **C.** true **D.** true **E.** true

In radionuclide imaging dose increases in proportion to:

- the activity administered
- the effective half-life of the radionuclide

$$\frac{1}{\text{Effective half-life}} = \frac{1}{\text{biological half-life}} + \frac{1}{\text{physical half-life}}$$

- the energy of the radiation emitted
- the emission yield (or percentage emission of γ-rays per disintegration)

This varies between different nuclides.

A 25. **A.** true   **B.** false   **C.** true   **D.** false   **E.** true

Spatial resolution is the ability to distinguish two objects. It is improved by:

- decreasing slice thickness
- increasing matrix size
- decreasing pixel size
- reducing the field of view

Below a certain pixel size, spatial resolution is further limited by the size of the focal spot, collimators, number and size of detectors, and spacing between the detectors. Low contrast spatial resolution is limited by the noise in the image.

Question	A	B	C	D	E
1	T	T	F	F	T
2	F	T	F	F	F
3	F	T	T	T	F
4	F	T	F	T	F
5	F	T	F	F	F
6	T	T	F	T	F
7	F	T	T	T	F
8	T	T	T	F	F
9	F	F	T	F	T
10	T	T	T	T	F
11	F	F	T	T	F
12	F	F	T	F	F
13	T	F	T	F	F
14	F	T	F	F	T
15	F	T	F	T	F
16	T	F	F	F	T
17	F	F	F	T	T
18	F	T	F	T	T
19	F	T	T	T	F
20	F	F	F	T	T
21	T	T	F	F	F
22	F	F	F	T	F
23	F	F	T	T	F
24	T	F	T	T	T
25	T	F	T	F	T

A 1. **A.** true **B.** true **C.** false **D.** false **E.** true

The valence electron is in the outer shell.

The atomic number (Z) is the number of protons in the nucleus.

The mass number (A) is the total number of protons and neutrons in the nucleus, i.e. the number of nucleons. In a non-ionised atom, the number of protons equals the number of orbital electrons.

A 2. **A.** true **B.** true **C.** false **D.** true **E.** false

X-rays have a shorter wavelength than visible light and hence a higher frequency. Electromagnetic radiation (EMR) does not include particulate emission from radioactive decay. It is impossible to distinguish between two wave packets (or quanta) of EMR of the same energy, as to whether they are from an X-ray or a γ-ray source.

Electromagnetic radiation energy per photon (keV) = 1.24/wavelength (in nm). Auger electrons are not EMR.

A 3. **A.** false **B.** true **C.** true **D.** false **E.** true

A stationary anode tube is not used with a high kV because of the build-up of heat in the system. However some low tube potential techniques may still require rotating anode technology, such as in mammography.

Output of the tube is proportional to mA and kV².

Rotating anodes are made of a tungsten-rhenium alloy as it improves the thermal capacity of the anode and resists roughening.

The efficiency of X-ray production is 1% (99% of electron-electron interactions produce heat).

A 4. **A.** false **B.** true **C.** true **D.** true **E.** false

Output is decreased by an increase in filtration as the lower energy X-rays are filtered out preferentially to higher energy ones. However, the overall intensity at all photon energies is reduced.

Output is proportional to kV² and mA.

The anode material will affect the yield of X-rays produced.

Output is unrelated to focal spot size (for the same target angle).

A 5. **A.** true **B.** true **C.** false **D.** true **E.** true

Intensity is the total amount of energy per unit area passing through a cross section per unit time. It is also called the energy fluence rate at that point.

It is dependent on tube current.

It is dependent on the atomic number of the target material and is proportional to atomic number Z.

The radiation intensity follows an exponential attenuation law when passing through a material:

$$I(x) = I(o) \cdot e^{-\mu x}$$

where μ is the linear attenuation coefficient, x is the thickness of tissue and I(o) = the incident intensity.

According to the inverse square law, the intensity of the radiation is inversely proportional to the square of the distance from a point source.

A. true **B.** false **C.** false **D.** true **E.** true

The aim of filtration is to remove a large proportion of the lower energy photons before they reach the skin. This reduces the dose received by the patient while hardly affecting the radiation reaching the film, and so the resulting image.

It is usually made of aluminium for general diagnostic tubes.

National standards require that the total filtration is not less than 2.5 mm Al for general X-ray tubes, 1.5 mm for dental units operating below 70 kVp and not less than 0.03 mm molybdenum for mammography units.

A. true **B.** false **C.** true **D.** true **E.** true

Half value layer (HVL) is the thickness of a stated material that will reduce the intensity of a narrow beam of X-radiation to half its original value.

$HVL = 0.69/\mu$ where μ is the linear attenuation coefficient which measures the attenuating properties of the material and is the fraction of the primary beam removed per unit distance.

The photoelectric effect predominates over the Compton interaction in high atomic number materials, e.g. in bone below 50 keV, and in soft tissue below 30 keV.

In soft tissue the characteristic radiation produced is very low energy that it is absorbed locally.

The probability of the Compton effect (Compton linear attenuation coefficient, σ) decreases only slightly with increasing energy over the photon energies used in diagnostic radiology.

The Compton effect predominates in CT because of the higher energy photons used compared to general X-ray.

Examination Three

Answers

A 8. **A.** false **B.** false **C.** false **D.** false **E.** true

Reducing the X-ray field size reduces the volume of scattering tissue and so decreases scatter.

An air gap technique results in a large reduction in the intensity of the scattered radiation reaching the film/screen, this is typically a 30 cm gap.

For diagnostic X-ray beams the scatter distribution from Compton interactions is very approximately uniform in space, i.e. is not heavily forward peaked. The measured scattered dose distribution from a patient shows a higher dose on the entrance side due to absorption in the patient of forward scattered radiation.

A 9. **A.** true **B.** false **C.** false **D.** false **E.** false

In mammography, single coated films are used.

The focal spot is smaller, 0.3 mm or less.

The X-ray tube has a molybdenum target and is used at 28 kVp with a molybdenum filter. Other combinations, such as rhodium, are also available and can be useful for thicker breasts and a higher kV technique.

The heel effect is helpful when the chest wall is placed nearer the cathode, where the beam is more intense.

A 10. **A.** true **B.** false **C.** true **D.** true **E.** false

Output is measured with an electronic kV meter. Output is proportional to kV^2.

'Leeds' test objects are used to test image quality and require the subjective assessment of images of various test objects.

Focal spot size can be measured with a pinhole camera or star test object.

For standard radiographic installations one would normally expect the measured value to be within ±5 kV or 5% of the nominal value. It is usually recommended that errors of 10 kV or more be corrected before further use. Mammography equipment is subject to tighter controls.

A **11.** **A.** true   **B.** false   **C.** false   **D.** true   **E.** true

Decreasing the kVp results in an increase in mAs to maintain a constant receptor dose, which gives rise to film blackening, resulting in an increase in patient dose.

An aluminium filter attenuates the lower energy X-rays more in proportion to the high energy X-rays, reducing skin dose to the patient without affecting the image.

A compression band reduces the thickness of tissue irradiated.

Grids reduce scatter reaching the film; they result in an increase in dose to the patient as a greater mAs are required for the same exposure. Low ratio grids are less selective. So they will allow more scatter to reach the film, but will allow exposure factors to be reduced.

A **12.** **A.** false   **B.** false   **C.** true   **D.** false   **E.** true

Stochastic effects are assumed to be a linear function of dose with no threshold dose.

The probability of the effect occurring (rather than its severity) increases with dose.

Stochastic effects induce cancer.

A **13.** **A.** false   **B.** false   **C.** false   **D.** false   **E.** false

For stochastic effects, the probability of an effect occurring (not its severity) increases with dose. Whereas for deterministic effects, once a threshold is exceeded, the severity of the effect increases with dose.

The equivalent dose (mSv) is the absorbed dose (mGy) multiplied by the radiation weighting factor for the radiation used. The dose equivalent is a previous definition of radiation dose by the International Commission on Radiological Protection and is not mentioned in the regulations. It is similar in definition to equivalent dose but should not be used.

A classified worker is a member of staff who has been classified a radiation worker, and they require statutory health and radiation monitoring.

Local rules specify the procedures needed to ensure compliance with the law. They cover safety organisation, descriptions of controlled areas, and the systems of work for working in the controlled areas and for restricting access to them.

A 14. A. false   **B.** true   **C.** true   **D.** true   **E.** true

Absorbed dose, measured in Gy is the amount of energy imparted per unit mass to a medium by the incident radiation.

Equivalent dose, measured in Sv, is the product of the absorbed dose and a radiation weighting factor (w_R). This is because the same organ dose will not produce the same biological effects if the radiation type is different.

Radiation type	Radiation weighting factor (W_R)
X-rays, γ-rays, and electrons	1
Protons	5
Alpha particle	20
Neutrons	5–20

Equivalent dose is combined with the tissue weighting factor to calculate effective dose E, also in Sv. It is not averaged over different organ types but weighted with a weighting factor w_T.

A 15. **A.** true   **B.** true   **C.** false   **D.** false   **E.** false

Air has an effective atomic number (7.6) close to that of soft tissue (7.4). In an unsealed air chamber the pressure and temperature will affect the number of gas molecules in the chamber and can affect the reading. In diagnostic radiology dosimetry an error of a few percent may be acceptable in the context of other errors.

In radiotherapy a correction will have to be taken into account. Free air chambers are housed in national standards laboratories; they are some 800 times the size of thimble chambers. IRR (1999) does not specify how dose is measured, but the quantities measured have to conform to international standards of measurement and quantities.

A 16. **A.** false   **B.** true   **C.** false   **D.** false   **E.** true

Effective dose limit is 1 mSv to a member of the public.

The limit on equivalent dose for the skin is 500 mSv averaged over any 1 cm² area regardless of the area exposed for employees, and 50 mSv for a member of the public, 13 mSv during any consecutive 3 month period to the abdomen of a woman of reproductive capacity.

The effective dose for an employee is 20 mSv per year, or 50 mSv in special circumstances where the employer demonstrates to the HSE that it cannot meet the 20 mSv/calendar year limit.

Body part	Dose limits (mSv)			
	Employees ≥18 years	Special circumstances	Trainees aged under 18 years	Other people (incl. <16 years)
Effective dose/year	20	50	6	1
Equivalent dose for skin/year	500	500	150	50
Equivalent dose for lens/year	150	150	50	15
Equivalent dose for abdomen of a women of reproductive capacity/3 m	13	13	N/A	N/A

A 17. **A.** false **B.** true **C.** false **D.** false **E.** true

According to IRR (1999) the dose limit for employees 18 years or over is 20 mSv. A controlled area is necessary where there is significant risk of spread of contamination, or where a person is likely to receive E >6 mSv or 3/10 of employee equivalent dose limit.

Patient doses to be as low as reasonably practicable (ALARP). There is no set limit they must be below.

A 18. **A.** false **B.** true **C.** false **D.** false **E.** false

Dose monitoring badges are ineffective at detecting surface contamination for which a contamination monitor is required. Scintillation crystal monitors are ideal for measuring personal contamination from electron capture or γ emitting nuclides.

Mouth pipetting is not permitted under any circumstances.

Following a spill decontamination should be carried out. This involves the use of water, mild detergents, and swabs which are then sealed in plastic bags and disposed of as radioactive waste in marked bins under an agreed waste disposal procedure.

Lead aprons are ineffective against the high-energy γ-rays of ^{99m}Tc and generally local shielding is much more effective at reducing dose rates.

A 19. A. true   **B.** true   **C.** true   **D.** true   **E.** true

Film speed is the reciprocal of the air kerma needed to produce D = 1, which is the average density of a properly exposed radiograph.

It is affected by:

- Photon energy of the X-rays (typically greatest at 30–40 keV)
- Presence or thickness of screen
- Atomic number of screen material
- Film grains: narrower, aligned grains are more likely to stop most of the X-rays compared to rounded grains

It is also affected by development effects

- Concentration of developer
- Developer temperature
- Development time

A 20. A. true   **B.** false   **C.** true   **D.** true   **E.** false

The shape of the characteristic curve is largely determined by the properties of the film because of the range of grain sizes affecting γ.

The saturation density cannot normally be exceeded as it is a fixed level dependent on the properties of the film. At very high doses reversal can happen however. High kV techniques reduce subject contrast enabling the effective latitude of the images to be increased.

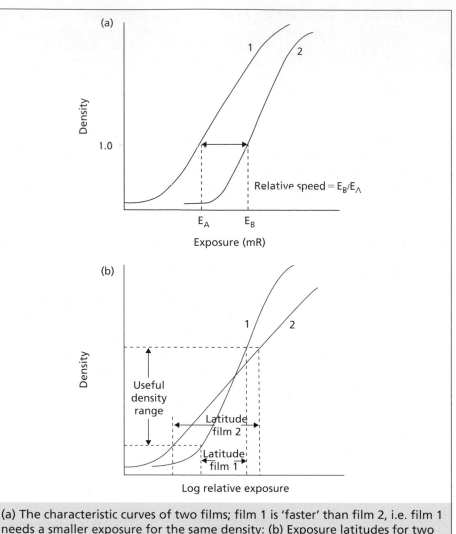

(a) The characteristic curves of two films; film 1 is 'faster' than film 2, i.e. film 1 needs a smaller exposure for the same density: (b) Exposure latitudes for two medical X-ray films; film 2 has a lower contrast than film 1 but has a wider latitude.

A fast screen, using phosphor with a high X-ray to light conversion efficiency, requires a lower X-ray dose or exposure (fewer photons/mm^2) and give a worse signal to noise ratio.

A 21. **A.** true **B.** true **C.** false **D.** true **E.** false

Efficiency of the crystal is dependent on its thickness. It is hygroscopic so must be sealed in a container.

The size of the pulse from the photomultiplier tube is proportional to the original γ-ray energy.

Gamma rays can not be focused. Instead of a lens, a multihole collimator is used to delineate the image from the patient. The primary function of the collimator is therefore not to reduce scatter.

A 22. **A.** false **B.** true **C.** true **D.** true **E.** false

The activity of 1 Bq = 1 disintegration per second.

In transient equilibrium the daughter decays as quickly as it is formed. Such that the daughter and parent decay together with the half-life of the parent. If the half-life of the daughter is shorter than the parent, then in equilibrium the activity of the daughter present is

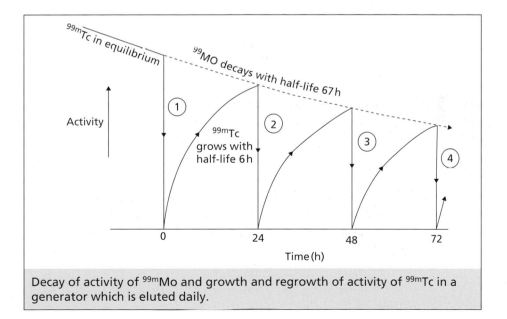

Decay of activity of ^{99m}Mo and growth and regrowth of activity of ^{99m}Tc in a generator which is eluted daily.

independent of its own half-life. The amount of daughter present decays exponentially with the activity of the parent.

Activity is related to the time between elutions as it takes time for the amount of daughter to regenerate after each elution.

A **23.** **A.** false   **B.** false   **C.** false   **D.** true   **E.** true

When the daughter is in transient equilibrium with the parent nuclide, the daughter is decaying as fast as it is being formed. The daughter and parent decay together (i.e. same activity) with the half-life of the parent. After elution, the daughter nuclide decays at its own half-life. At the same time more daughter is being formed from the parent. After 24 h the activity has grown again to a new maximum (equilibrium) for a Mo99/Tc99m generator. By definition if parent and daughter are in equilibrium then the time since last elution is irrelevant, however the amount of daughter present will depend on the time since the last elution.

A **24.** **A.** true   **B.** true   **C.** false   **D.** true   **E.** false

Modulation transfer function (MTF) measures:

$$\frac{\text{Information in the image}}{\text{Information in the object}}$$

Every imaging system suffers from loss of information and so has a MTF. It is affected by any aspect of imaging that can result in a blurred image.

It is used to:

- Compare imaging systems
- Assess deterioration in performance of a system
- Measure the MTF of each separate component of an imaging system

A. true   **B.** true   **C.** false   **D.** true   **E.** false

The brightness or grey scale value of each pixel represents the average linear attenuation coefficient of the contents of the corresponding voxel.

Nearly all CT is operated at a kVp of 140, at these high energies Compton interactions predominate in the patient.

A 'bow-tie' filter is used providing a filtration equivalent to 0.5 mm of copper.

Narrowing of the window width increases contrast as it allows small differences of CT number to be selected from the full range and displayed over the whole grey scale.

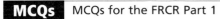

Question	A	B	C	D	E
1	T	T	F	F	T
2	T	T	F	T	F
3	F	T	T	F	T
4	F	T	T	T	F
5	T	T	F	T	T
6	T	F	F	T	T
7	T	F	T	T	T
8	F	F	F	F	T
9	T	F	F	F	F
10	T	F	T	T	F
11	T	F	F	T	T
12	F	F	T	F	T
13	F	F	F	F	F
14	F	T	T	T	T
15	T	T	F	F	F
16	F	T	F	F	T
17	F	T	F	F	T
18	F	T	F	F	F
19	T	T	T	T	T
20	T	F	T	T	F
21	T	T	F	T	F
22	F	T	T	T	F
23	F	F	F	T	T
24	T	T	F	T	F
25	T	T	F	T	F

A 1.   **A.** true   **B.** true   **C.** true   **D.** true   **E.** true

In β decay an electron is ejected from the nucleus with high energy and is called a β− particle. There is no change in mass number, but the atomic number increases by one. As a β particle passes through tissue it causes ionisations and excitations of atoms in the material along its track until it has lost all of its energy. The total range involved in tissue interactions is a few millimetres at most, but in air up to a few metres. The range of β particles from phosphorus 32 is up to 6 m in air.

A 2.   **A.** true   **B.** false   **C.** true   **D.** false   **E.** true

A molybdenum filter transmits most of the characteristic radiation but removes most of the continuous spectrum of a molybdenum target. A lot of low energy photons are produced at the target via bremsstrahlung, but they are almost all filtered by the tube housing, glass wall and added filtration.

The focusing cup acts to prevent the electron stream from spreading and striking the target over a large area which would otherwise lead to blurring.

A 3.   **A.** true   **B.** false   **C.** false   **D.** true   **E.** false

If an X-ray tube is operated below the K absorption edge of the target anode material no characteristic radiation is produced, i.e. K_α or K_β lines cannot be seen in the X-ray spectrum. However, the spectrum still shows the continuous bremsstrahlung shape always evident with an X-ray spectrum and is therefore not monoenergetic.

Even using a K-edge target and filter, other portions of the X-ray spectrum are still evident, although reduced. Some mobile image intensifier X-ray systems utilise rotating anode X-ray tubes.

The maximum current density falling on the target anode puts limitations on the tube current and focal spot size. Hence, the number of X-ray photons per mm² will be constant for both fine and broad focus. A large focus is used for thicker parts of the body that require a greater intensity of X-rays (and hence a higher tube current) in order to keep exposure times acceptably short. Smaller focal spots give better resolution, but at the expense of lower tube current and longer exposure times. X-ray tube life depends on its workload history and how it has been used, but is not accurately predictable. It is possible to get several years work out of a typical busy X-ray tube. Mobiles do not require high speed tubes because of tube loading.

A 4. **A.** true **B.** false **C.** false **D.** false **E.** false

The amount of scatter reaching the film may be reduced, and contrast increased, by putting a grid between the patient and the film. Using a grid requires an increase in the mAs, increasing the dose to the patient from primary and scattered radiation.

A 5. **A.** false **B.** false **C.** false **D.** true **E.** true

Increasing filtration:

- increases the penetrating power (HVL) of the X-ray beam
- increases the minimum and effective photon energies but does not affect the maximum photon energy
- reduces the area under the energy fluence spectrum and the total output of X-rays
- increases the exit dose/entry dose ratio or film dose/entrance surface dose ratio

A. false **B.** true **C.** false **D.** false **E.** false

Film-screen combinations do not affect scatter around the patient. Measures to reduce the amount of scatter produced by the patient include:

- reducing the field size
- compression of the patient
- lowering the kV

Increased filtration leads to beam hardening, which increases average photon energy in the spectrum. This tends to increase the proportion of Compton interactions taking place out of the total number of interactions. Scattered photons may have high enough energy to escape the body thus giving rise to a scatter dose in the vicinity of the patient. In this case the beam intensity was reduced by the additional filtration and the X-ray factors kept the same. Of the remaining photons it is certainly true that a greater proportion of them will be Compton scattered, however their overall total number has been reduced. Therefore the scatter dose is lower than the unfiltered case.

Increasing the focus skin distance has the effect of increasing the area irradiated on the patient but does not change the total number of photons reaching the patient. The scatter will therefore be the same. Increasing the object to film distance (i.e. an air gap) reduces scatter to the film leaving the scatter from the patient unchanged. At diagnostic X-ray exposures measured scatter doses are greater on the entrance side, i.e. backward scatter, due to absorption of the forward scattered beam in the patient.

A 7. **A.** true **B.** true **C.** false **D.** false **E.** false

Effective focal spot size is determined by:

- the target angle
- the actual focal spot size, which in turn is determined by:
  - the size of the filament; and
  - the presence of a focusing hood

A 8. **A.** true **B.** false **C.** true **D.** false **E.** true

In the air gap technique the film is moved 30 cm away from the patient so that much of the wide angled scatter misses the film. The technique requires an increase in kV or mAs. A wide latitude low γ film-screen combination is required for chest radiography enabling the range of 'exposure' between bones, mediastinum and lung in the thorax to be captured on the film. Often a high kV is used to reduce subject contrast therefore reducing the required latitude of the film/screen combination.

A 9. **A.** false **B.** false **C.** true **D.** true **E.** false

For magnification of suspicious lesions, 0.1 mm focal spots are used. Rhodium or even palladium can be used as beam filter materials with higher kVs for thicker breasts. As well as reducing dose, compression immobilises the breast (exposure times are quite long), reduces object film distance (reducing film blurring) and equalises tissue thickness. Here the anode heel effect is useful and the thicker part of the breast can be positioned towards the cathode where the exit beam is more intense. A very fine moving grid is used to improve contrast.

A **10. A.** false   **B.** false   **C.** true   **D.** false   **E.** true

The film screen dose is proportional to $kV^4 \times mAs$. $80^4/60^4 = 3.16$. Therefore to achieve the same image receptor dose (related to film blackening), the mAs need to be cut to 32% of its previous value. A higher kV increases the penetration of the beam (fewer photoelectric interactions) and reduces patient dose. A lower kV increases film contrast.

A **11. A.** false   **B.** false   **C.** true   **D.** false   **E.** true

The intensity of an X-ray beam is:

- proportional to kV^2
- greater for a constant potential than a pulsating potential
- proportional to the mA
- decreased as the filtration is increased
- inversely proportional to the square of the distance from the target
- greater for higher atomic number targets than lower atomic number ones

It falls inversely as the square of the distance.

A **12. A.** true   **B.** false   **C.** false   **D.** false   **E.** false

Blurring is reduced by:

- using a smaller focal spot
- decreasing the object-film distance
- or using a longer film focus distance which also reduces magnification and distortion

Movement blurring may be reduced by immobilisation and by using a short exposure time. However, this is not counted as geometrical unsharpness.

A 13. **A.** false   **B.** false   **C.** false   **D.** false   **E.** false

Grid ratio is the height of the lead strips divided by the distance between them. Grid factor is the exposure necessary with a grid divided by the exposure necessary without it. Primary transmission is the measure of the tendency of the grid to reduce primary radiation and is of the order of 70%.

A 14. **A.** false   **B.** true   **C.** false   **D.** true   **E.** true

The effects have been demonstrated with exposure to radiation.

A 15. **A.** true   **B.** true   **C.** false   **D.** false   **E.** false

When X- or γ-rays are absorbed by thermoluminescent (TL) material, atomic electrons are raised to higher energy levels and stay in their excited state ('electron traps') indefinitely. TL material can be made in a range of sizes allowing measurement of finger and eye doses, for example. Precision of 1% is only achievable with electronic dosimeters. TLDs do require calibration. Processing of TLD can involve heating up to 300–400°C.

A 16. **A.** false   **B.** true   **C.** false   **D.** false   **E.** true

The larger the number of X-ray photons absorbed the less quantum mottle. Only using a longer exposure time or exposing a film twice, increases the number of photons absorbed on a film. The use of screens increases quantum mottle because fewer photons are needed for the same film blackness.

A 17. **A.** false   **B.** true   **C.** false   **D.** false   **E.** true

Fog is the density of processed but unexposed film. Inherent fog is due to some of the silver bromide crystals having acquired latent images during manufacture, and the film base absorbing light when viewed. Additional fog may arise from:

- Increasing film age
- Incorrect storage (high temperature and humidity)
- Increasing developer temperature/time
- Accidental exposure to X-rays
- High film speed

A **18. A.** true   **B.** true   **C.** false   **D.** false   **E.** false

The steps of film processing are:

I. Developing: Immersion in an alkaline solution of a reducing agent (pH 9.6–10.6) to reduce silver ions to silver atoms. If the temperature is too high, the reducing agent will start to react with non-ionised grains forming a background image, increasing fog.
II. Washing.
III. Fixation by an acid solution (pH 4.2–4.9) of thiosulphate which removes unaffected silver ions. The fixer contains aluminium salts which harden the film and reduce the drying time.
IV. Washing: The results of inadequate washing are that any retained thiosulphate turns brown/yellow.
V. Drying.

Film speed, γ and fog are affected by:

- Concentration of developer
- Developer temperature
- Development time

A **19. A.** false   **B.** true   **C.** false   **D.** true   **E.** true

The image intensifier at the output phosphor has a spatial resolution of 4–5 lp/mm. Veiling glare, due to the scattering of light, reduces contrast and is worse with the larger sizes of intensifier. Magnification increases input dose to retain the same output brightness. Quantum mottle (noise) is particularly noticeable in fluoroscopy unlike in radiography. Dose rates on the input surface of the image intensifier are of the order of $0.5\,\mu Gys^{-1}$ in fluoroscopy; the typical skin dose may be around 300 times greater.

A 20. A. true   **B.** false   **C.** false   **D.** false   **E.** true

Protective clothing does not protect against the direct beam, only radiation attenuated or scattered by the patient.

Aprons have a lead equivalent of 0.25 to 0.5 mm.

A 0.25 mm thick lead apron transmits less than 10% of 90° scatter for a 100 kVp scattered beam.

A 21. A. false   **B.** true   **C.** false   **D.** false   **E.** false

Under IRR (1999) an employee must become a classified worker if three-tenths of a dose limit are exceeded. In the case of the lens of the eye this is 30% of 150 mSv or 45 mSv per annum. Different employers are required to co-operate with dose monitoring under IRR (1999) but there is no absolute necessity to make shared workers classified.

A 22. A. false   **B.** false   **C.** true   **D.** true   **E.** false

Referrers are registered medical or dental practitioners, or other health professionals who are entitled to refer patients for medical exposure to a practitioner. Entitlement is a local decision. Employers need procedures for identifying all referrers. The practitioner and operator needs to be adequately trained; not the referrer.

A. false   **B.** true   **C.** true   **D.** true   **E.** false

Notify the Health and Safety Executive (HSE) of:

- dose exceeding dose limit
- medical exposure much greater than intended
- loss or theft of source
- release or spillage leading to a significant contamination

Internal reporting of:

- dose exceeding investigation level
- failure to follow work instructions and local rules
- near misses

A. true   **B.** false   **C.** true   **D.** false   **E.** false

The absorbed dose delivered to an organ increases in proportion to:

- the activity administered to the patient
- the effective half-life in the organ
- the energy of β and γ radiation emitted in each disintegration

The maximum usual dose of a Thallium-201 myocardial scan is approximately 18 mSv.

The dose delivered by a radionuclide examination is unaffected by the number of images taken.

A. true   **B.** false   **C.** false   **D.** false   **E.** false

The dose increases with the number of slices. By increasing the spacing, fewer slices will be imaged.

Dose is proportional to mA.

Increasing the number of detectors has no effect on dose.

In spiral scanning the dose depends very much on the scan protocol and it does not always follow that doses will be lower. However in long acquisitions tube loading may be a limitation and a lower mA may be used resulting in a lower patient dose.

As each slice needs to be reconstructed by all the ray paths available through the volume, all the detectors need to be used even with a smaller selected field of view (FOV). Hence selecting a smaller FOV will not affect the dose.

Question	A	B	C	D	E
1	T	T	T	T	T
2	T	F	T	F	T
3	T	F	F	T	F
4	T	F	F	F	F
5	F	F	F	T	T
6	F	T	F	F	F
7	T	T	F	F	F
8	T	F	T	F	T
9	F	F	T	T	F
10	F	F	T	F	T
11	F	F	T	F	T
12	T	F	F	F	F
13	F	F	F	F	F
14	F	T	F	T	T
15	T	T	F	F	F
16	F	T	F	F	T
17	F	T	F	F	T
18	T	T	F	F	F
19	F	T	F	T	T
20	T	F	F	F	T
21	F	T	F	F	F
22	F	F	T	T	F
23	F	T	T	T	F
24	T	F	T	F	F
25	T	F	F	F	F

A 1.   **A.** false   **B.** false   **C.** false   **D.** true   **E.** true

The Compton effect is an interaction between a photon and a free electron. The nature of the interaction is a process governed by probability. So for any given photon it is impossible to say through what angle and into what direction it may scatter. However, there is a scattering probability distribution that depends on the energy of the incident photon. For photons in a typical diagnostic energy spectrum the distribution is only slightly forward peaked. On average higher energy photons will scatter through a smaller angle than lower energy photons, and this effect predominates more the greater the initial energy of the photon. Greater the scatter angle of the photon greater the energy and the range of the recoil electron and greater the loss of energy (and increase of wavelength) of the scattered photon.

In the diagnostic X-ray energy range the fractional loss of energy of the incident photon is relatively small. For a 100 keV photon scattered through 60° the scattered photon has 91 keV of energy, and for an initial 30 keV photon the scattered photon has an energy of 29 keV.

The probability that a Compton interaction will occur is proportional to the electron density of the material. The electron density in electrons cm^{-3} is proportional to the physical density in gcm^{-3} multiplied by the number of electrons per gram which is given by NZ/A, where N is Avogadro's number and Z/A is the ratio of atomic number to mass number.

A 2. **A.** true   **B.** true   **C.** false   **D.** true   **E.** false

The Z of lead is 82. The Z of aluminium is 13, whereas the effective value for bone is 13.8. The photoelectric effect is important with high atomic number elements according to the following equation:

The photoelectric coefficient is proportional to $\rho Z^3/E^3$.

No scatter is produced although the process may result in characteristic X-rays being produced or the emission of Auger electrons. The photoelectric effect is about 45 times more likely in a given thickness of lead compared to aluminium.

The Compton effect predominates in CT because a high kV (120–140) is used and the beam is heavily filtered to increase the average spectral energy.

A 3. **A.** true   **B.** true   **C.** false   **D.** true   **E.** false

The Compton process is more important than photoelectric absorption with low Z materials above about 30 keV (e.g. fat has a Z of 6).

The photon only gives up some of its energy as kinetic energy to the recoil electron in Compton scatter.

The probability of the Compton interaction is proportional to density, and independent of Z.

A 4. **A.** true   **B.** true   **C.** false   **D.** true   **E.** true

Scatter is the result of Compton interactions.

It is increased with:

- increased subject thickness
- increased field size
- increased kV

Using a low kV produces less scatter and so, less reaches the film.

Scatter is reduced by:

- collimation
- grids
- air-gaps
- compression

Scattered radiation is uniform over an image, and acts like a veil reducing the contrast that would otherwise be produced by the primary radiation.

At the energy levels used in radiography, the highest scatter dose rates are at the entrance side of the patient due to backscatter. Attenuation in the forward direction reduces the scatter measured on the exit beam side of the patient. Therefore, overcouch tube units lead to larger staff eye and thyroid doses because the scattered dose rates are greater than a corresponding undercouch tube system.

A 5. **A.** true **B.** false **C.** true **D.** true **E.** false

HVL decreases as:

- the density of the material increases
- the atomic number of the material increases
- as the photon energy of the radiation decreases

Air-equivalent material absorbs energy from an X-ray beam to the same extent as a mass of air.

The output of an X-ray tube depends on the:

- kV
- mA
- filtration
- the target material
- kV waveform

A larger ion chamber measures the dose in a larger volume of air. Neglecting geometry effects, the dose (energy absorbed per unit mass) in air will be the same for both chambers irrespective of chamber size. Larger chambers can measure lower dose rates as they have a larger collection volume and are more sensitive.

A 6. **A.** false **B.** true **C.** false **D.** true **E.** false

The intensity of an X-ray beam is proportional to kV². A higher kV reduces the mAs needed to expose a radiograph to a given optical density because (a) the output per mAs is greater for a given mAs value and (b) the beam is more penetrating. As the mAs required is reduced, exposure times may be reduced also. High kV reduces skin dose as the beam is more penetrating, and the ratio of exit to entrance surface dose is increased. Using a higher kV produces slightly more forward and more penetrating scatter.

A 7. **A.** false **B.** false **C.** false **D.** false **E.** true

Collimation of the X-ray beam:

- decreases scatter
- reduces dose to the patient
- increases contrast

A 8. **A.** false **B.** true **C.** true **D.** false **E.** false

Contrast is improved by:

- reducing the field size
- compression of the patient
- reducing the kV
- using a grid
- using an air-gap
- using a filter placed on the cassette

A 9. **A.** true **B.** false **C.** false **D.** true **E.** false

Geometrical unsharpness is reduced by:

- using a small focal spot
- decreasing the object-film distance

- using a longer focus film distance
- using a longer focus object distance

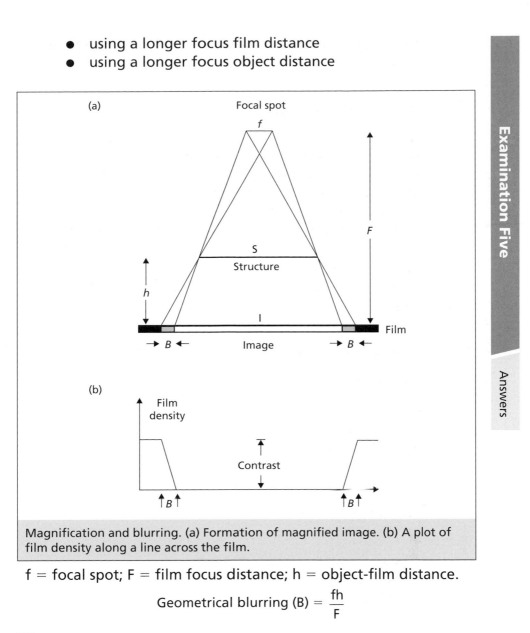

(a) Focal spot

Magnification and blurring. (a) Formation of magnified image. (b) A plot of film density along a line across the film.

f = focal spot; F = film focus distance; h = object-film distance.

$$\text{Geometrical blurring (B)} = \frac{fh}{F}$$

A 10. **A.** true **B.** true **C.** false **D.** false **E.** false

High kV (in excess of 100 kVp):

- increases the penetration of the beam
- reduces patient dose
- increases the latitude of exposure and the range of tissues displayed

- reduces the mAs needed allowing shorter exposure times
- reduces contrast

High kV techniques are used in chest radiography, radiography of the lumbar and dorsal spine, fluoroscopy of the gastro-intestinal (GI) tract, and in CT.

A **11.** **A.** false   **B.** false   **C.** false   **D.** true   **E.** false

Scatter produced by the patient, is reduced by reducing the field size, and compression of the patient. The proportion of scatter to primary beam does not depend on the speed of the film screen combination, or the tube current selected. Decreasing the tube filtration, will soften the beam and reduce the amount of scatter but also drives up patient dose.

A **12.** **A.** true   **B.** false   **C.** true   **D.** true   **E.** false

$$\text{Radiographic contrast} = \text{film } \gamma \times \text{subject contrast}$$

Subject contrast depends on:

- the thickness of the structure
- subject density
- atomic number Z
- kV

Film γ depends on the range of grain sizes (not their average size).

A **13.** **A.** true   **B.** false   **C.** false   **D.** true   **E.** true

The IRR (1999) dose limit for members of the public is 1 mSv per annum.

The average annual background radiation dose is 2.2 mSv per annum in the south-east of UK or approximately 6 μSv per day.

Entrance surface dose is defined as the absorbed dose to air at the point of intersection of the X-ray beam axis with the entrance surface of the patient, including back scattered radiation. For a chest radiograph it is around 0.2 mGy.

An 800 MBq SPECT bone scan gives an effective dose of 5 mSv.

A **14.** **A.** false **B.** true **C.** true **D.** false **E.** true

Some dose saving equipment:

- fast film screen combinations
- low attenuation (e.g. carbon fibre) materials for cassette fronts, grid interspacing, and table tops
- constant potential generators with appropriate kV
- appropriate beam filtration (at least 2.5 mm Al for general radiography)
- a pulsed digital fluoroscopy system at low pulse rates
- a digital fluoroscopy acquisition system reduces the need for film radiographs
- dose-area product meter to measure patient exposure

Magnification with the image intensifier makes the image less bright, necessitating an increase in exposure factors to compensate for the smaller minification gain on the smaller field of view (FOV). The area of anatomy exposed will be reduced in size, however one would expect an examination carried out on smaller FOV to require more screening and more digital radiographs to complete the examination thus giving a greater patient dose.

A **15.** **A.** true **B.** true **C.** true **D.** true **E.** false

The responsibilities of the employer are:

- Risk assessment
- Exposure restriction
- Area designation

- Training
- Monitoring
- Quality assurance of procedures

A **16.** **A.** false   **B.** false   **C.** true   **D.** false   **E.** false

The Radiation Protection Supervisor is needed to supervise work in areas where local rules are required. They are trained in:

- Nature of radiation and its effects
- Principles of restriction of exposure
- Quantities used
- Measurement techniques
- Legal requirements
- Principles of radiation protection
- Local knowledge

The Radiation Protection Adviser investigates overexposures.

A **17.** **A.** false   **B.** false   **C.** true   **D.** false   **E.** true

The employer has overall responsibility for keeping the dose as low as reasonably practicable (ALARP).

A **18.** **A.** false   **B.** false   **C.** false   **D.** true   **E.** true

The crystals of an intensifying screen absorb X-rays and emit light. Speed depends on the photon energy of the X-rays.

$$\text{Speed} = \frac{1}{(\text{Air kerma at } D = 1)}$$

Lanthanum oxybromide activated with the rare earth terbium, emits a line spectrum of blue light. Gadolinium oxysulfide emits 540 nm photons in the green portion of the spectrum, and is also activated using terbium. Rare earth screens have a lower K-edge absorption energy

Examination Five

Answers

(La$_2$OBr is 39 keV, Gd$_2$O$_2$S is 50 keV) than calcium tungstate screens (70 keV). Consequently they absorb radiation strongly just above these energies that lie close to the peak of the X-ray spectrum. Therefore, rare earth screens' response does depend on tube potential.

A 19. **A.** true   **B.** false   **C.** false   **D.** true   **E.** true

A film exposed with screens is more sensitive than the same film exposed without screens. The use of screens reduces the exposure needed, and the dose to the patient. The use of screens increases γ from about 2 to 3.

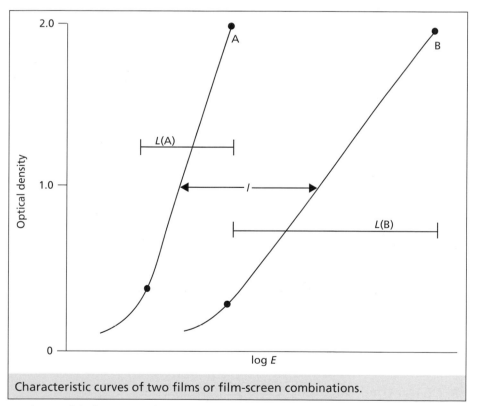

Characteristic curves of two films or film-screen combinations.

A has a higher γ and narrower latitude L(A).
B has a lower γ and wider latitude L(B).

A **20.** **A.** true   **B.** false   **C.** true   **D.** false   **E.** true

Rare earth screens are more efficient at converting X-rays into the light that exposes the film. For each X-ray photon, they produce a greater yield of light photons. Also thicker screens convert a greater proportion of incident X-ray photons into light. Consequently, fewer incident X-ray photons are needed to give the film the required level of exposure. Hence, the greater quantum noise (or mottle) seen with rare earth screens and thicker screens, is actually a result of their greater dose efficiency.

A **21.** **A.** false   **B.** true   **C.** false   **D.** true   **E.** false

The overall spatial resolution is worse than 1 lp/mm.

The pulse height analyser rejects pulses which are outside a preset range, to reduce the contribution of scattered radiation to the image. In some cases more than one energy window level is set, for instance to increase sensitivity with a multi-energetic radionuclide, or to create two separate images of different radionuclides present at the same time (e.g. V/Q scans and parathyroid imaging).

Intrinsic spatial resolution can be improved by using a thinner crystal.

The photoelectric effect predominates in the crystal at 140 keV photons, forming the photopeak.

A collimator locates a radioactive source along its line of sight, without it no image would be formed.

A **22.** **A.** true   **B.** false   **C.** false   **D.** true   **E.** true

Technetium has a γ energy of 140 keV. Its half-life is 6 h. ^{99m}Tc decays by isomeric transition to ^{99}Tc with the emission of a γ-ray. ^{99m}Tc and ^{99}Tc are isomers: nuclei having different energy states but otherwise indistinguishable as regards mass number, atomic number, numbers of protons, neutrons and other properties. Technetium 99m is the daughter of Molybdenum 99, and is produced from it in a generator.

Fluorine 18 is used in positron emission tomography (PET) imaging and decays by positron emission with a half-life of 110 min and is produced in a cyclotron.

A **23. A.** false   **B.** true   **C.** true   **D.** false   **E.** false

Gamma camera collimators can be changed for different purposes, but not the crystal. Contrast resolution can only be improved at the expense of either increased patient dose or worsened spatial resolution. The spatial resolution of a γ camera collimator is worse when the distance from the face of the collimator is increased, and when the holes of the collimator are wider or shorter. In tomography (e.g. SPECT) spatial resolution is worse than in conventional γ imaging, but contrast resolution is improved. A radionuclide should emit γ-rays of energy 50–300 keV and ideally of 150 keV, high enough to exit the patient but low enough to be easily collimated and easily measured.

A **24. A.** true   **B.** true   **C.** true   **D.** false   **E.** false

High spatial resolution imaging involves increasing the matrix size or reducing the field of view, thus decreasing the pixel size.

Noise in CT may be reduced by increasing the number of photons absorbed in each voxel, by increasing slice thickness, or the pixel size.

Ionisation chambers are less sensitive than scintillators.

The Compton process predominates in CT.

A. true   **B.** false   **C.** true   **D.** false   **E.** true

In CT spatial resolution improves with increasing matrix size. It is much poorer than plain radiography.

Tiny calcifications are made visible because of partial volume averaging, as a high contrast object occupying only part of a voxel will raise the CT number for the corresponding pixel and so give rise to image contrast.

Noise may be reduced by increasing the slice thickness.

The larger the object we are trying to detect the greater the number of pixels over which the noise can be averaged and better the signal to noise ratio.

Question	A	B	C	D	E
1	F	F	F	T	T
2	T	T	F	T	F
3	T	T	F	T	F
4	T	T	F	T	T
5	T	F	T	T	F
6	F	T	F	T	F
7	F	F	F	F	T
8	F	T	T	F	F
9	T	F	F	T	F
10	T	T	F	F	F
11	F	F	F	T	F
12	T	F	T	T	F
13	T	F	F	T	T
14	F	T	T	F	T
15	T	T	T	T	F
16	F	F	T	F	F
17	F	F	T	F	T
18	F	F	F	T	T
19	T	F	F	T	T
20	T	F	T	F	T
21	F	T	F	T	F
22	T	F	F	T	T
23	F	T	T	F	F
24	T	T	T	F	F
25	T	F	T	F	T

Examination Five

Answers

A 1. **A.** true **B.** true **C.** false **D.** true **E.** true

The mass number (A) is the total number of protons and neutrons in the nucleus.

The atomic number (Z) is the number of protons in the nucleus. This is constant and determines the chemical characteristics of the element. The nucleus is formed of protons and neutrons. It is 10^{-15} m in diameter. It is concerned with the production of radioactivity (γ-rays).

Compton scattering involves a free electron not the nucleus. An atom is excited when an electron is raised from one shell to another further out.

A 2. **A.** true **B.** false **C.** true **D.** false **E.** false

All the photon energy is absorbed.

The photoelectric effect is important at low energy levels (mammography) and with high Z elements: PE effect is proportional to $\rho Z^3/E^3$.

The K-edge of lead is at 88 keV.

The photoelectric effect is more likely to occur in bone because of its higher Z number.

A 3. **A.** false **B.** true **C.** true **D.** true **E.** false

In diagnostic X-ray production only 1% of the energy used is converted into ionising radiation, 99% of it is converted to heat. This target heating is a limiting factor. Two methods are implemented in the design of an X-ray tube to overcome this.

Line focus principle

The target is tilted. The target angle θ is the angle between the central ray and the target face. Electrons are focused on an area of the target AB. This is the 'actual focal spot', the area over which heat is produced and which determines the tube rating. Because the target is tilted, the 'effective focal spot' BC, is shortened in one direction.

This technique produces a small focal spot but can dissipate heat over a large area.

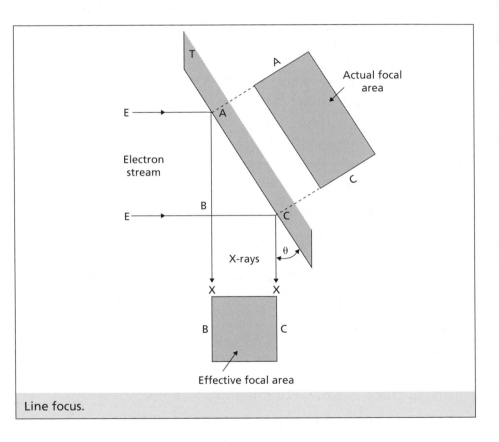

Line focus.

Rotating anode tube

Rotating the anode also increases the area over which the heat is produced and helps to dissipate it.

Anode heel effect – Intensity of beam is lower on anode side of field, as radiation has to transverse the longer edge of the bevelled anode.

A 4.   **A.** true   **B.** false   **C.** true   **D.** false   **E.** true

The heat rating of an X-ray tube is usually stated as the allowable mA. It:

- decreases as exposure time is lengthened
- decreases as the kV is increased, in inverse proportion
- increases with the effective focal spot size, and for a given effective focal spot size, is greater for smaller target angles
- is greater for a rotating than stationary anode
- is greater for a high speed anode
- is greater for a three-phase constant potential than a pulsating potential

A 5.   **A.** false   **B.** true   **C.** true   **D.** true   **E.** false

In high kV techniques:

- subject contrast is low
- skin dose is reduced
- efficiency of X-ray production is high. This reduces heat loading and allows shorter exposure times
- scattered radiation is high, reducing the effectiveness of grids
- air gap technique is preferred

A 6.   **A.** true   **B.** true   **C.** false   **D.** true   **E.** false

Secondary electrons refer to the recoil electrons of Compton scatter, and the photoelectrons of the photoelectric effect.

A 7. **A.** true **B.** false **C.** false **D.** true **E.** true

In mammography:

- Compression is always used unless it is not tolerated or there is an open wound.
- The molybdenum filter preferentially allows the characteristic radiation of the molybdenum target through.

A 8. **A.** false **B.** true **C.** false **D.** true **E.** true

The air gap is between the film and the patient.

The air gap technique produces a magnified image.

In CT, collimators in front of the detectors are used to reduce scatter, and the air gap reduces scatter dose as well.

A 9. **A.** false **B.** false **C.** true **D.** true **E.** true

Cancer induction is a stochastic process and has a linear response. There is no threshold.

Severity increases with dose in deterministic effects, not stochastic ones.

A 10. **A.** false **B.** false **C.** false **D.** true **E.** false

Some dose saving techniques:

- use non-grid techniques when examining children
- use the largest practicable focus to skin distance
- a large focal spot reduces exposure time but not patient dose
- fast film-screen combinations
- high kV technique as less energy is deposited in the patient

A 11. **A.** true   **B.** true   **C.** false   **D.** true   **E.** false

The threshold for skin erythema is about 2 Gy.

Cataracts of the lens are produced above threshold of about 5 Gy.

There is little or no risk to the live born child from irradiation during the first 3 weeks of gestation. From 3 to 8 weeks since conception there is a potential for the malformation of organs. From 8 to 25 weeks, there is a potential for severe mental retardation. From 4 weeks to term, there is the potential for cancer in childhood and adult life.

X-rays, γ-rays and electrons have the same radiation weighting factor.

A 12. **A.** true   **B.** true   **C.** true   **D.** true   **E.** false

Use of a constant potential waveform means the spectrum corresponds to that kV value and is not changing to lower values during an alternating mains cycle. The average kV is greater and the beam more penetrating. Hence patient doses will be lower.

A 13. **A.** false   **B.** true   **C.** true   **D.** true   **E.** false

Employees likely to receive dose greater than 6 mSv or 3/10 of employee equivalent dose limits will be designated a classified worker.

A 14. **A.** true   **B.** true   **C.** false   **D.** false   **E.** false

In a supervised area a person is likely to receive an effective dose >1 mSv or >1/10 of employee equivalent dose limit.

In a controlled area a person is likely to receive an effective dose >6 mSv or >3/10 of employee equivalent dose limit.

15. **A.** true **B.** true **C.** true **D.** false **E.** false

A diagnostic reference level (DRL) is a dose level, or amount of radioactivity used in a diagnostic procedure for typical examinations. It is not a dose limit.

Each hospital sets its own DRL; this should be compared with the national one. DRLs can be assessed using skin dose level, kV, mAs, dose product, or screening time.

Different DRLs are set for different age ranges in paediatrics.

DRLs are not normally exceeded under standard conditions.

16. **A.** true **B.** false **C.** false **D.** true **E.** false

The DAP meter is mounted on the light beam diaphragm.

Effective dose is the sum of the weighted equivalent doses for all the tissues that have been exposed, and has to be calculated.

The HSE must be informed if the exposure is between three and twenty times the dose intended depending on the examination being performed.

17. **A.** false **B.** false **C.** true **D.** true **E.** true

Gamma is the steepness of the characteristic curve and is related to film contrast.

It is dependent on grain size in film emulsion and range of grain size, as well as processing factors (e.g. concentration of developer, developer temperature, development time).

18. **A.** false **B.** true **C.** false **D.** false **E.** false

Screen unsharpness is light diffusion within the screen phosphor layer. It is worse with faster screens as the phosphor layer is thicker.

A 19. **A.** false **B.** false **C.** false **D.** true **E.** true

The input screen is made of caesium iodide and is 170 mm or more in diameter.

The caesium-antimony photocathode converts the light into electrons.

The resolution of smaller details is improved if the field of view is smaller.

The brightness gain = flux gain × minification gain
(50 − 100) × (100 − 200)

The output screen is typically 25 mm in diameter.

A 20. **A.** false **B.** false **C.** true **D.** true **E.** false

The crystal thickness cannot be changed readily, but collimators can. Non-uniformity can be attributed more to the variations in photomultiplier tube response than the crystal.

The crystal is fragile and must be protected from physical and thermal shock and moisture.

A narrower window width centred on the spectrum photopeak reduces the count rate coming into the system, but also discriminates against scattered photons being included in the image.

Gamma rays cannot be focused, so a multihole collimator is used to delineate the image from the patient.

A 21. **A.** false **B.** true **C.** false **D.** false **E.** true

^{99m}Tc is the daughter product of ^{99}Mo, is produced in a generator and has a γ energy of 140 keV. It decays by isomeric transition to ^{99}Tc which is radioactive and has a half-life of 200,000 years.

A 22. **A.** true **B.** false **C.** false **D.** false **E.** true

The ideal radionuclide:

- is a pure γ emitter
- is easily made
- localises largely and quickly in the area of interest
- emit γ-rays ideally about 150 keV
- has a physical half-life of a few hours

Lead aprons are ineffective against high energy γ-rays.

Radioactive waste can be disposed of by containment and decay, or by dilution. Gases can be vented to the air. Liquid waste can be diluted and sluiced direct to the foul drain. Solid waste can be incinerated or sent to landfills.

Patients containing radioactivity are a source of radiation. They should be spaced apart in the waiting area.

A 23. **A.** true **B.** true **C.** true **D.** false **E.** false

A water phantom is used in CT to measure image uniformity.

Focal spot can be measured with a star pattern or a pinhole camera.

Leeds test objects are subjective checks of image quality. They check:

- grey scale
- low contrast detectability
- minimum visible detail
- uniformity of focus
- image size and distortion

An ion chamber and electrometer measures dose, not exposure time.

The tube potential can be measured with a penetrameter or kV dividers.

24. A. false **B.** true **C.** false **D.** true **E.** true

The Hounsfield unit for fat is around −100.

$$\text{The CT number of a pixel} = 1{,}000(\mu_t - \mu_w)/\mu_w$$

w = water; t = tissue.

The Compton effect is more important than photoelectric absorption, with higher energy photons.

Spatial resolution improves with increasing matrix size or reducing the field of view, thus decreasing pixel size, but at the expense of increased noise.

Using a narrower window width makes noise more noticeable, as each grey level covers a smaller range of CT numbers. However, contrast in the displayed range improves contrast and visibility.

25. A. false **B.** false **C.** false **D.** true **E.** true

Collimators at the detectors:

- Control scattered radiation
- Regulate the thickness of the slice

To compensate for the diminishing patient thickness towards the edges of the fan beam a 'bow tie' filter is used.

High specification tubes are used in all CT applications.

Examination Six

Answers

Answers

Question	A	B	C	D	E
1	T	T	F	T	T
2	T	F	T	F	F
3	F	T	T	T	F
4	T	F	T	F	T
5	F	T	T	T	F
6	T	T	F	T	F
7	T	F	F	T	T
8	F	T	F	T	T
9	F	F	T	T	T
10	F	F	F	T	F
11	T	T	F	T	F
12	T	T	T	T	F
13	F	T	T	T	F
14	T	T	F	F	F
15	T	T	T	F	F
16	T	F	F	T	F
17	F	F	T	T	T
18	F	T	F	F	F
19	F	F	F	T	T
20	F	F	T	T	F
21	F	T	F	F	T
22	T	F	F	F	T
23	T	T	T	F	F
24	F	T	F	T	T
25	F	F	F	T	T

A 1.   **A.** true   **B.** false   **C.** true   **D.** true   **E.** false

The range increases with an increase in the initial energy of the particle. The exact relationship is complex but very approximately proportional. Lighter particles have longer ranges than heavier particles of the same energy and charge. Lower the charge, further the particle travels. A particle with half the charge travels four times the distance. Higher the density, shorter will be the range. The relationship is very approximately linear.

A 2.   **A.** false   **B.** false   **C.** true   **D.** false   **E.** true

Compton collisions occur when a photon interacts with free electrons. They produce a scattered photon and a recoil electron. The probability of a Compton interaction occurring is proportional to the physical density of the material. It is independent of the atomic number of the material, as it concerns only free electrons.

In the diagnostic energy ranges up to 20% of the energy is absorbed, the rest being scattered.

A 3.   **A.** true   **B.** false   **C.** true   **D.** true   **E.** false

In a Compton interaction a photon interacts with a free electron which recoils taking away energy from the photon. The photon is scattered with reduced energy. The angle of scatter is the angle between the scattered ray and the incident ray. Greater the angle of scatter, lower the energy of the scattered photon.

A 4. **A.** false **B.** false **C.** false **D.** true **E.** true

Characteristic radiation is produced when a filament electron collides with a K-shell electron of the target material, ejecting it and causing an electron to fall into the K-shell from the L-shell. This results in the emission of a single X-ray photon of energy equal to the difference in the binding energies of the two shells.

It is characteristic of the target material.

A 5. **A.** false **B.** false **C.** false **D.** false **E.** false

The inherent filtration is equivalent to 0.5–1 mm of Al and is produced by the following components:

- Window of the tube housing
- Insulating oil
- Glass insert
- The target itself

A beryllium window may be used instead of glass, when inherent filtration must be minimised as in mammography.

The total filtration is the sum of the added filtration and the inherent filtration. This is equivalent to 2.5 mm of Al.

It is responsible for absorbing low energy X-rays with long wavelengths.

A 6. **A.** false **B.** false **C.** true **D.** false **E.** true

The binding energy of an electron is the energy required to completely remove it from an atom against the attractive force of the positive nucleus. The kinetic energy is the energy it gains when it escapes.

The binding energy is expressed in electronvolts (eV). It is dependent on the shell (increasing the nearer the shell is to the nucleus) and the atomic number, increasing as Z increases.

A 7. **A.** true **B.** true **C.** false **D.** false **E.** false

The target forms part of the anode which is the positive electrode.

Tungsten is suitable due to its high atomic number and high melting point.

The Auger electron is produced by the absorption of the characteristic radiation emitted by the photoelectric effect in biological materials.

Because Wavelength = 1.24/Energy, the minimum wavelength of the X-ray depends on the kVp.

The effective focal spot remains the same. The rotation of the target is aimed to dissipate heat.

A 8. **A.** true **B.** true **C.** false **D.** true **E.** true

The quality of an X-ray beam depends on:

- kVp, since a higher kVp produces a beam of higher average energy
- Rectification, since this determines the kV variation with time
- Filtration, since a filter is used to 'harden' the beam

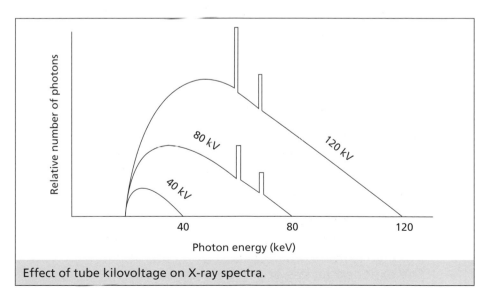

Effect of tube kilovoltage on X-ray spectra.

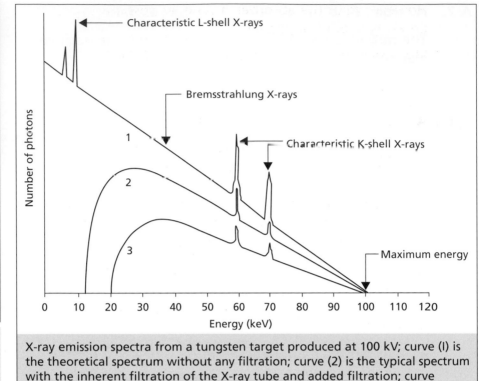

X-ray emission spectra from a tungsten target produced at 100 kV; curve (1) is the theoretical spectrum without any filtration; curve (2) is the typical spectrum with the inherent filtration of the X-ray tube and added filtration; curve (3) shows the effect of added filtration.

A 9. **A.** false **B.** false **C.** false **D.** true **E.** false

Exponential X-ray attenuation is where equal thicknesses of an absorber transmit equal percentages of the radiation entering them.

The intensity of radiation is inversely proportional to the distance from a point source in the absence of scatter and absorption; this is the inverse square law.

The beam intensity would be decreased by a factor of 2^{10} (=1,024).

In a polyenergetic beam, as it passes through an attenuating material, lower energy photons are attenuated more than the higher energy ones.
The exponential law does not apply exactly.

However thick the absorber, it is never possible to absorb an X-ray beam completely.

The linear attenuation coefficient (μ) = 0.69/HVL.

A **10.** **A.** true   **B.** true   **C.** false   **D.** false   **E.** true

$$\frac{1}{\text{Effective half-life}} = \frac{1}{\text{biological half-life}} + \frac{1}{\text{physical half-life}}$$

Metastable isotopes involve the emission of a γ-ray but no other particle and it is due to a 're-arrangement' of the nucleon energy states in the nucleus.

Alpha decay is the emission of an α particle, which is a helium nucleus: 2 protons and 2 neutrons. The atomic number therefore decreases by 2, the mass number by 4.

A sheet of paper easily stops an α particle.

A **11.** **A.** false   **B.** true   **C.** false   **D.** true   **E.** false

The children of irradiated parents show no increase in the incidence of congenital defects or life expectancy. The genetic risks of irradiation are only theoretical and have not been proven statistically.

Damage to the lens of the eye is one of the highest deterministic risks and occurs above a threshold of about 5 Sv to the eye. Once a threshold is exceeded the severity of deterministic effects increases with dose.

The probability of stochastic effects occurring does increase with increased dose. The severity of stochastic effects is, however, independent of the dose.

Irradiation of the fetus at 3–8 weeks after conception carries the highest risk of organ malformation.

The weighted equivalent dose must first be derived by multiplying each organ dose by a weighting factor for that organ as described by the International Commission on Radiological Protection report (ICRP 60). The weighted equivalent doses are then summed up to give the effective dose.

A 12. **A.** true   **B.** false   **C.** false   **D.** true   **E.** true

Processing a thermoluminescent detector causes light to be emitted. The total light emitted (the area under the 'glow curve') is proportional to the dose of X- or γ-rays absorbed.

Electronic dosimeters allow direct reading of dose and rate.

Film badges have filters; the pattern of which gives an indication as to the type of radiation to which it has been exposed. TLDs cannot differentiate between energies unless several are combined in a dosimeter each having a different attenuating filter. However, the actual thermoluminescent material cannot give information on the radiation energy itself.

A 13. **A.** false   **B.** true   **C.** true   **D.** true   **E.** true

Absorbed dose is the energy absorbed from a beam of radiation per mass of material: Grays (Gy) are defined as Joules per kilogram.

The radiation weighting factor is an indication of the effectiveness of the radiation type compared with that of electrons in inducing cancers at low doses and low dose rates.

A **14.** **A.** false   **B.** false   **C.** true   **D.** true   **E.** false

The instantaneous dose rate on the outside of the shielding of equipment containing radioactive substance is kept ALARP however it may not necessarily have to be below 7.5 µSv per hour.

IRR (1999) does apply to radiation beam therapy and testing.

The employer is also bound to keep a report of any investigation for at least 2 years from the date in which it was made.

The regulations allow for trainees of less than 18 years of age. The dose limits for trainees of less than 18 years is, however, lower than those aged 18 and over.

A **15.** **A.** false   **B.** false   **C.** true   **D.** true   **E.** true

The effective dose combines organ doses to give a single whole body dose.

Gamma rays and X-rays have the same radiation weighting factor. Alpha particles are 10–20 times more damaging.

Because the radiation weighting factor is 1, equivalent dose is numerically equal to the absorbed dose in tissue, but are measured in different units (absorbed dose in mGy; equivalent dose in mSv).

The radiation weighting factor for α particles is 20, and for neutrons it varies between 5–20, depending on neutron energy.

A **16.** **A.** true   **B.** false   **C.** false   **D.** false   **E.** false

Equivalent dose for the lens of the eye in a year is 50 mSv for a trainee under 18 years of age.

Effective dose not equivalent dose in a year is 20 mSv.

Effective dose limit in a year to a member of the public is 1 mSv.

Equivalent dose to abdomen of a women of reproductive capacity at work, should not exceed 13 mSv in any consecutive three-month period. For pregnant workers, exposure should be restricted so that the fetal dose is unlikely to exceed 1 mSv for the remainder of the pregnancy (~2 mSv to abdomen).

A 17. A. false **B.** false **C.** false **D.** true **E.** true

A worker must be classified if the dose to an organ (e.g. their hands) exceeds 3/10 of the dose limit 500 mSv/year (i.e. 150 mSv). One course of solid bricks is roughly equivalent to 10 cm of high density concrete in terms of room protection.

A 18. A. true **B.** false **C.** true **D.** false **E.** false

The system is exposed to a series of exposures in predetermined steps so that the relationship between one exposure and another can be recorded and plotted against the densities produced on the film.

The characteristic curve is obtained by plotting the optical density not its log against log relative exposure.

Base density is due to an increased absorption of light as it is transmitted through the polyester film base.

Grain size and other film emulsion characteristics determined during manufacture such as grain distribution are important determining factors of the gradient.

The speed (or sensitivity) of a system is an expression of the exposure required to obtain a certain optical density. Higher speed is therefore obtained when the characteristic curve shifts to the left.

A 19. **A.** false **B.** true **C.** false **D.** true **E.** true

The emulsion crystals contain 10% iodide and 90% bromide. Each crystal is about 1 μm in size and contains more than a million silver atoms.

The light photons interact with the crystal to liberate electrons which migrate towards the sensitivity speck, attracting mobile silver ions which are then neutralised to produce a speck of silver metal at the site of the sensitivity speck. This is the latent image that will be used to form the final image in the development process.

The screen coating the posterior emulsion functions by absorbing X-rays transmitted through the anterior screen. Light photons produced by the anterior screen should be absorbed by the anterior emulsion and should not reach the posterior emulsion.

The agent in the development process should be an electron donor such that the positive silver ions are reduced into silver metal grains. This agent should be alkaline, unlike the fixing solution which should be acidic.

Increasing the developer temperature increases the rate of chemical reaction, increasing the speed of the film.

A 20. **A.** false **B.** true **C.** true **D.** false **E.** false

Film fog influences the final radiographic contrast but does not influence subject contrast.

Greater the density differences between different tissues, greater is the difference in the attenuation of the beam.

The photoelectric effect is the most important determinant of subject contrast in soft tissue radiography. Closer the kVp to the atomic numbers of the subject matter, higher the photoelectric attenuation, and hence higher the subject contrast.

This tends to increase the subject contrast by the photoelectric effect.

The total exposure affects the final blackening of the film and may affect radiographic contrast but does not influence subject contrast.

A 21. A. false   **B.** true   **C.** true   **D.** false   **E.** false

Caesium iodide is favoured because its absorption edges are more favourable and also its crystals are ideal for alignment with the X-ray beam and can be packed together more tightly increasing the efficiency of the screen.

The light produced at the input phosphor is immediately converted to electrons by the photocathode coating the phosphor, the light produced at the output phosphor is used to form the image on the camera, film or monitor.

The area of the input phosphor is larger than the area of the output phosphor by about 100 times. The ratio of the two is known as the minification gain which increases the brightness of the image.

The centre of the final image is brighter than the periphery of the image. This is due to the difficulty of controlling the peripheral electrons by the electron beam and due to vignetting in the optical lens system capturing the image at the output phosphor.

Magnification is typically produced by varying the voltages on the intermediate electrodes. The input dose to the image intensifier must be increased in order to retain the same brightness at the output phosphor of the intensifier when a magnified field of view is selected. Using a magnified field improves the resolution of the image. Image intensifier systems normally collimate the X-ray beam down to the magnified field of view.

A 22. **A.** true **B.** false **C.** false **D.** true **E.** false

The main purpose of a collimator is that γ-rays from a selected area of the organ reach a selected area of the crystal for improved spatial resolution. This is achieved by using collimators with different designs.

The resolution is decreased as the thickness of the crystal is increased.

The pulse height selector selects pulses that have the desired energy, to reduce the contribution of scatter to the image.

The flash of light the crystal emits, illuminates the array of photomultiplier tubes.

The main cause of variation in the image is electronic in nature.

A 23. **A.** true **B.** false **C.** false **D.** true **E.** true

The effective dose delivered by a radionuclide examination is unaffected by the number of images taken. Most investigations deliver an effective dose of 1 mSv or less.

The absorbed dose delivered to an organ (the energy deposited per unit mass) increases in proportion to:

- The activity administered to the patient
- The effective half-life of the activity in the organ
- The energy of β and γ radiation emitted in each disintegration

For a given study the administered activity is chosen to give the appropriate detected count rate at the γ camera.

A low energy nuclide has γ-rays that are less penetrating, i.e. more of them may be absorbed in the patient. In such cases increased activity must be given in order to retain an acceptable count rate at the camera.

For children the activity administered should be reduced because their smaller size and weight means that less γ-rays are absorbed and an acceptable count rate can be achieved at a lower administered activity.

A 24. **A.** false **B.** true **C.** false **D.** false **E.** false

The Hounsfield unit of each pixel is a weighted average of all the constituents of the voxel.

The presence of a very high attenuating material (e.g. calcium) will elevate the CT number of the entire pixel enabling something to be seen. This is partial volume averaging.

Nearly all CT is operated at a tube potential of 120–140 kVp. At these energy levels Compton interactions predominate.

A 25. **A.** false **B.** false **C.** false **D.** false **E.** false

Using a narrower window increases the effect of noise because each grey level would represent a smaller range of CT numbers.

A bow tie filter is used to aid the process of applying a beam hardening correction by compensating for the thinner patient thickness around the outside of the patient, i.e. the ray paths have to pass through less patient nearer the periphery of the field of view.

Increasing the slice thickness decreases the effect of noise because more photons are detected.

Line pair resolution is only about one line pair per mm and so is much poorer than that obtainable in film-screen radiography.

The phenomenon called cupping, an abnormally lower attenuation at the centre of the CT image, is caused by beam hardening as the X-ray beam passes through the patient. This artefact is compensated for by using compensatory algorithms.

The pitch of a helical scan is increased by increasing the speed of the table movement. This speeds up the scanning and reduces dose but greater interpolation is needed, thus reducing resolution.

Question	A	B	C	D	E
1	T	F	T	T	F
2	F	F	T	F	T
3	T	F	T	T	F
4	F	F	F	T	T
5	F	F	F	F	F
6	F	F	T	F	T
7	T	T	F	F	F
8	T	T	F	T	T
9	F	F	F	T	F
10	T	T	F	F	T
11	F	T	F	T	F
12	T	F	F	T	T
13	F	T	T	T	T
14	F	F	T	T	F
15	F	F	T	T	T
16	T	F	F	F	F
17	F	F	F	T	T
18	T	F	T	F	F
19	F	T	F	T	T
20	F	T	T	F	F
21	F	T	T	F	F
22	T	F	F	T	F
23	T	F	F	T	T
24	F	T	F	F	F
25	F	F	F	F	F